CW01023654

Sex,
Guys and
Chocolate

Other books by Dr Pam Spurr

Sinful Sex – The Uninhibited Guide to Erotic Pleasure
(Robson Books)
The Dating Survival Guide – The Top Ten Tactics for Total
Success (Robson Books)
The Break-up Survival Kit – Emotional Rescue for the Newly
Single (Robson Books)
Understanding Your Child's Dreams (Sterling Publishers NY)
Dreams and Sexuality – Interpreting Your Sexual Dreams
(Sterling Publishers NY)

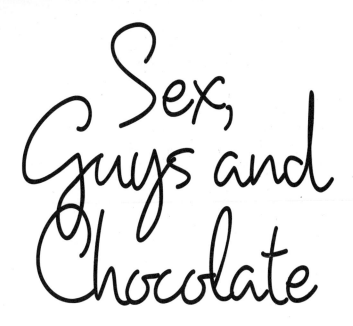

Sex, Guys and Chocolate

Your Essential Guide to
Lust, Love and Life

Dr Pam Spurr

ROBSON
BOOKS

In memory of my terrific parents – Arthur and Winifred
For Nick – ever supportive of me
For Sam and Stephie – my precious treasures

First published in Great Britain in 2003 by Robson Books,
The Chrysalis Building, Bramley Road, London, W10 6SP

An imprint of Chrysalis Books Group plc

Copyright © 2003 Dr Pam Spurr

The right of Dr Pam Spurr to be identified as the author of this work has
been asserted by her in accordance with the Copyright, Designs and
Patents Act 1988.

The author has made every reasonable effort to contact all copyright
holders. Any errors that may have occurred are inadvertent and anyone
who for any reason has not been contacted is invited to write to the
publishers so that a full acknowledgement may be made in subsequent
editions of this work.

British Library Cataloguing in Publication Data
A catalogue record for this title is available from the British Library.

ISBN 1 86105 691 5

All rights reserved. No part of this publication may be reproduced, stored
in a retrieval system, or transmitted in any form or by any means,
electronic, mechanical, photocopying, recording or otherwise, without
the prior permission in writing of the publishers.

Typeset by SX Composing DTP, Rayleigh, Essex
Printed by Butler & Tanner Ltd, London and Frome

While every effort has been made to ensure that the information is
correct at the time of going to press, the information in this book is for
information only. It is not intended as a substitute for the advice and
guidance of a qualified health professional. If in doubt, seek medical
advice.

Neither the author nor the publisher can accept responsibility for any
accident, injury or damage that results from using the ideas, information
or advice offered in this book.

Contents

Acknowledgements

I'd like to thank every person who has helped me with *Sex, Guys and Chocolate* by sharing their life stories with me. When someone asks another person for advice this becomes a two-way process: by asking, hopefully they get something helpful from the process; but at the same time, they open the eyes of the person *giving* advice. I love talking to people about their stories because that is what life is about – each individual's story. What we forget is that we *are* the authors of our own stories. So be creative and powerful when writing yours! . . . Lastly, warm thanks to my publisher, Jeremy Robson.

Introduction

I'm continually asked for a handy little guide to life. Yes – *life*! Tall order! We've all become so used to easy access to information on the Internet that women now want the next logical step – a book that contains a little bit of everything. Even on the Internet you often have to trail from site to site looking for what you want, and we're not always within reach of a computer when we want some information, motivation or inspiration – so writing this guide seemed to make complete sense.

We are now so busy that creating a book you can quickly flip through for lots of answers seemed a fantastic project to get involved with, and one close to my heart as my work has covered so many aspects of women's problems. Please note that I say '*lots* of answers', as no single book can contain *all* the answers to the dilemmas we face in modern life when the rules seem to change all the time. But hopefully you'll find plenty of useful advice and inspiration within the following chapters, and suggestions that may become a springboard to sorting out other matters.

How did I decide what to include? As my work as a life coach, agony aunt and psychologist has covered such a range of different areas, it made sense to have a good look at what most women ask about, where they get stuck, and the most common problems they face. Trawling through literally thousands of e-mails, letters and queries I've received in recent years pointed me in the right direction.

As I looked through all these women's queries it dawned on me that they fell roughly into three areas: 'lust' (sex), 'love' (guys) and 'life' (chocolate). These are the essential areas about which most women have questions, even if they chat about them with their friends and family. Often we simply want an unbiased opinion and a constructive attitude from someone who is neutral – and that's where I've come in over the years in my various roles.

When it comes to sex – lust – we're in a bit of a muddle. In fact we're in more than a muddle – men *and* women are downright confused! Who does what to whom? Where's my sex drive hiding? Why is my sex life so boring? Many of our attitudes to sex have changed but too often we don't have the knowledge to keep up with the changes. This leads to women feeling a lack of confidence about what they want from sexual relationships. But questions such as 'when should I have sex?' and 'do men prefer oral sex to penetration?' are not the only kinds I'm asked in this area. Women want to know more about STIs (sexually transmitted infections), new sexual techniques, Tantric and safer sex, among many other things.

In terms of guys – love – we get so many mixed messages nowadays that I've taken some crucial issues and provided straightforward advice and information supported by psychological research into relationships. We worry about being independent, then we are concerned we can't form healthy relationships, and we wonder why we end up in unhappy cycles of relationships. We're not even sure what we want. I hope you can find in my advice the inspiration and information you need to improve your chances of finding and keeping love.

In the chapter called 'Chocolate', I've provided some essential guidance to help you make the most of your life. People constantly ask me why they feel empty, drained and worthless; why they feel unfulfilled while living in the wealthiest generation ever. Women also want to know how they can identify their good points, put them to use, develop skills and move forward. So much of general happiness with life is about attaining balance in its many facets. It's about being motivated and getting on and also about not overlooking the little stuff – the simple joys that we can treasure each day. Two pieces of advice I received from my parents put this in perspective. Shortly before my mother passed away in January 2003 she said to me, 'Be as happy as you can be.' My father said to me before his passing in May 1999, 'Grab opportunities with both hands!' Two very different pieces of advice but nonetheless related. When you're at your happiest you're most likely to grab those opportunities. And when you grab opportunities you'll feel happy. All of life is interlinked in this way.

If you don't find the answer to your particular dilemma in these pages then please take a closer look at some of the organisations I've mentioned, which may offer further information. Also I hope that some topics will provide food for thought. At the time of writing the phone numbers and websites listed in this book were accurate.

Good luck with your adventures in lust, love and life! We only have one shot – make yours the best you can!

SEX —
Lust

Why Do You Want Sex Anyway?

Can you answer the question, 'Why do you want to have sex anyway?' Right now you may be wondering why I'm asking *you* that! 'Because I want to feel good Dr Pam – Doh!' Well let me tell you that women have sex for completely different reasons. Because they want physical closeness, because they want to be loved, because they're drunk or high on drugs, because they get an emotional 'high' from it, because they've been pressured into it, because they want something and they think sex may lead to it, for revenge, because they're chasing an elusive orgasm and hope to get it this time, because they simply think they should – as a young liberated woman, among many other reasons.

One of the most important rules for having good sex is knowing why you're getting into bed with someone – because this helps prevent regrets. If you've thought this far about having sex then you're more likely to go to bed with someone for the right reasons. Or at least you may know you're on a path to nowhere if your reasons are dodgy. Forewarned is forearmed. Here are some *good* reasons to have sex:

- ✓ You're in lust and confident – so you're not worried if it ends up as a one-night stand.
- ✓ You're falling for someone and now it seems right.
- ✓ You're in love and he is too.
- ✓ You've a busy life and simply need sexual gratification on your terms – and he knows what they are – no strings attached. 'Bonk buddies' – as it's called!

All of these examples and other reasons are fine – *if they're fine for you* and you practise safer sex.

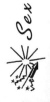

Play Safer!

The sexiest lovers are those who care about their sexual health – *and* that of their lover. They don't want to catch or spread sexually transmitted infections (STIs). Any potential lover you come across who will *not* use condoms is *a* simply not sexy. And *b* no one you should have sex with. In an ideal world – rather than the real world we inhabit – both of you will have condom confidence. Just in case you come across a man who doesn't feel comfortable putting on a condom – build your own condom confidence. Get a variety *free* from your GP family planning clinic, local GUM (genito-urinary medicine) clinic, or any other birth control agency. *Read the instructions first!* Open the packet carefully so that you don't damage the condom. Grip the tip of the condom to squeeze out any air. Slide it on to a vibrator, carrot, cucumber, broom handle – anything penis shaped! Voilà – it's that easy. Practice makes perfect! Male condom complaints:

❖ 'I can't feel anything with a condom.' **Solution** Put a drop of water-based lube inside the tip of the condom to enhance his sensations, and try the 'extra-sensitive' types.

❖ 'I can't find a condom that fits.' **Solution** Try the huge variety available – there's one for every penis shape!

❖ 'I want to really *feel* you!' **Solution** Both get screened for STIs, then retested for human immunodeficiency virus (HIV) – then go for it without condoms. It'll feel *even better* once you've waited!

❖ 'Condoms irritate me!' **Solution** Use ones without Nonoxynol-9 (N-9), the spermicide that irritates some people. Many specialists in sexual health, such as the National AIDS Trust, are asking for the removal of N-9 from condoms and lubricants as it's now believed it *increases* the risk of HIV infection. However, its use in spermicidal creams and gels for use with other forms of barrier contraception (sponges, pessaries, etc.) is considered safe for women at low risk of HIV infection, i.e. in relationships with men they can trust.

Safer Sex — Talking About It

You deserve sexual health so how do you start talking about it? Here are points to consider smoothing any communication along.

Where Research shows that talking about sex in the bedroom can make matters worse. The reason? If the conversation takes a negative turn, a couple may then associate the bedroom with a negative experience, clouding future sexual encounters there. Always having sex in the bedroom can get boring – but bed-sex has its place. Most people make love in their bedroom or sitting room. So choose neutral ground. Also, if you start getting hot and horny in the bedroom you may not finish the conversation!

When It is always best to talk about sex when you're not heavily under the influence of alcohol (or drugs). Alcohol loosens our inhibitions and sometimes we may say things we regret or *in a way* we regret without enough tact. Of course, a little alcohol can relax you – and that's fine.

How Keep it simple – begin with, for example, 'I want to protect myself *and you* so I want to have safer sex.' If you beat about the bush your lover will think you have something to hide, or just get nervous about the whole thing if he lacks sexual confidence. You make it *easier* taking this approach. Always use a clear but relaxed tone of voice. Then simply ask, 'How do you feel about this?'

Finally If you agree, bring on the condoms! You'll already have condom confidence if you followed the previous advice above!

5

Preventing Sexually Transmitted Infections

So you know how to use condoms – but how do you get sorted and find out more about safer sex? Find out where your local GUM clinic is through your nearest hospital or GP or visit www.ruthinking.co.uk and search under 'Local Help'. There are also many private ones listed under 'clinics' in the Yellow Pages. They tend to keep standard office hours, but this does vary, so ring in advance. You'll be seen confidentially there (even your GP doesn't get informed unless you give permission) and the staff are specially trained in the field of sexual health and will answer *all* your questions. You could not ask for a better environment to find out about sexual health and screening for STIs. You may also have cervical smear tests, counselling and testing for HIV, as well as other services. So don't worry – just get yourself down there.

You don't need a referral or to book an advance appointment. If the clinic is busy you may have to wait. Some STIs can be diagnosed at the time through 'on the spot' tests. For others you'll have to come back or telephone for your results. GUM clinics see people who work in the sex industry – so nothing will shock them! The latest statistics from GUM clinics – previously called venereal disease (VD) or 'clap' clinics – across the country show STIs have more than doubled between 1995 and 2000. They continue to increase. In 2000, the number of new cases of gonorrhoea being diagnosed leapt to over 20,000, with chlamydia surging to 64,000 new cases and infectious syphilis to over 300 new cases that year.

Some STI Info To Get You Thinking

These are just a few of the nasties you might pick up.

Chlamydia A bacterium that can lay dormant for years. Symptoms include abdominal pain and vaginal discharge, among others. Scary fact – 70 per cent of women are symptomless.

Gonorrhoea Another nasty bacterium, taking two to ten days to show symptoms, including vaginal discharge, abdominal pain, painful urination – but over 60 per cent of women are symptomless.

Herpes Simplex Virus 1 and 2 HSV1 usually affects the mouth (cold sores) but sometimes the genitals, and HSV2 is the other way round. Oral sex can transmit it. You'll experience painful little clear or yellowish genital blisters. Recurrent attacks become less painful but it's a life-long problem. Treatment alleviates symptoms and you will be taught how to avoid passing the virus on.

Human Papilloma Virus (HPV) This causes genital warts, which can take months to show. They may appear as 'lumpiness' in the skin or as little 'cauliflower' style warts. There are different treatments available.

Syphilis Also known as the 'pox', this is a spiral-shaped germ that can take from one to twelve weeks to show. There are three stages. First, a painless red spot appears, becoming ulcer like. Then you may get a skin rash and, eventually, if left untreated, leads to, for example, blindness and heart problems.

Other STIs These include hepatitis, cystitis, bacterial vaginosis, balanitis, non-specific urethritis, pelvic inflammatory disease, lice, thrush, trichomonas and others. Any symptom you experience in the genitals, abdomen, and/or anal passage should be checked, as symptoms vary tremendously from person to person. Permanent damage to reproduction as well as death (syphilis) can result from leaving STIs untreated.

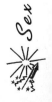

HIV And AIDS

The human immunodeficiency virus (HIV) multiplies within a person, living off the 'host' and preventing normal function of the white blood cells that help fight infections. HIV is passed on via any exchange of body fluids, including during sex, sharing needles among drug users, and in infected breast milk. Many who worry about their sexual health probably worry about HIV infection most because of its association with its development into full-blown acquired immune deficiency syndrome (AIDS), where the body can no longer fight the variety of infections we run into in daily life. The safer sex campaigns of the eighties did lots to raise awareness but now many people seem much less concerned.

The disease is still out there and it can take three to six months for an HIV test to register an antibody reaction in your system. As there are no specific symptoms for an HIV-positive person, the disease can go undetected for as much as ten or fifteen years. And, of course, it can be passed around during this time. The first indication of infection may be when a person has difficulty fighting off minor illnesses.

If you're HIV-positive, your doctor will more than likely prescribe anti-viral drugs, along with other medicines to help you fight off minor illnesses. Overall, doctors will help plan how to keep you healthy. There are other implications, too, which will be talked through at the GUM clinic. There are a number of sources of support for those diagnosed with HIV and/or AIDS. Ring the Sexual Health and National AIDS Help Line (0800-374-318) for further information.

Contraception

Successful contraception is only possible if used *as directed*. Contraception failures tend to occur when women don't follow instructions *to the letter*. You can get contraceptive advice at any Family Planning or reproductive health clinic, as well as from most GPs and some GUMs, at specific times. There are a number of clinics aimed especially at young people, such as the Brook Centres, for those aged under 25 (Help Line: 020-7617-8000).

Contraception allows you to take control of your life and decide when (if ever) you want to have a baby. There is a wide range of contraceptive products available. When you go for a consultation you should have a full and frank discussion of your sexual health and lifestyle needs. Ask any question you wish. It's advisable to go along with a question list so you don't forget anything. Even if you are under sixteen, Family Planning Clinics offer confidential advice and free contraception.

The range of contraception available includes the 'pill' or combined oral contraceptive; the 'mini-pill' containing progesterone only; female and male condoms; the diaphragm, which fits inside the vagina and is held in place by a spring; the cervical cap, which fits snugly over the cervix itself; IUDs (intra-uterine devices), which fit inside the cervix and prevent egg implantation; a combined system with an IUD that releases hormones; Norplant implants, lasting five years – which need specialist consultation; injectable contraception; emergency contraception, when you're worried about contraceptive failure such as a split condom, or have had unprotected sex (the 'morning after' pill may prevent pregnancy for up to 72 hours, while the IUD protects up to five days later); and male and female sterilisation. Contraceptive Education Service Help Line: 0845-310-1334.

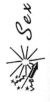

Conception — Making Mini-Yous!

Before you even start thinking about having sex *to have a baby* you should consider what creating a mini-you actually means! Many go into parenthood with rose-coloured specs on thinking how wonderful it'll be to have a baby to *love them!* It's quite the reverse – babies need your love and attention a full 24/7. There's no respite unless you've got parents or friends to help.

You and your partner should think about the changes a baby will mean to your relationship. No more lie-ins or late nights, or making love when you want. Go into it having agreed what sorts of roles you two will play. But be prepared for these to be thrown to the wind once you actually become parents. Do lots of babysitting for others to give you a small taster.

Aside from these practical and emotional considerations, look at your health and lifestyle – especially the mum-to-be. If you're actually planning a pregnancy – rather than having found yourself pregnant – consult your doctor or practice nurse about how long you should wait after coming off birth control before trying for a baby. For example, you may be advised to wait three months to clear your system of any hormones. Start taking a folic acid supplement (400 mcg daily until the twelfth week of pregnancy), stop smoking (more on this in Part Three: 'Chocolate – Life'!) and cut down on alcohol and caffeine in-take in preparation for a healthy pregnancy. Check out the National Childbirth Trust website (www.nctpregnancyandbabycare.com) for loads of info.

Termination

Terminating (aborting) a pregnancy is something you may or may not have to consider at some point. The most important thing, if you find yourself pregnant and it's unplanned, is to seek help so you can talk through your options. The longer you leave seeking help, the more difficult your choice may be. If you leave your pregnancy longer than 24 weeks you will not qualify for a termination.

At the present time, the abortion laws in the UK state that a woman may have an abortion up to 24 weeks of pregnancy. However, 90 per cent of abortions occur within the first 12 weeks of pregnancy. Only 1.2 per cent of abortions take place between 20 and 24 weeks. Abortion is not 'on demand' as two doctors must confirm a woman meets the criteria for abortion (for example, that she'd suffer mental distress if she did not have one). Doctors may refuse to carry out an abortion due to reasons of conscience. In that case they're obliged to refer you to another doctor who will. In later pregnancy, abortions are approved if they pose less risk to the mother's life than if the woman continued with the pregnancy.

At present, the question of whether you'll be eligible for a free NHS abortion varies from area to area. If you don't wish to go to your own doctor, there are a number of alternatives. For example, the British Pregnancy Advisory Service (0845-730-4030), a privately run charity, provides termination advice. Ring them or visit their website (www.bpas.org). Presently, an abortion arranged through such a service costs from £355 to £405, depending on your area.

The Look Of Lust – How To Tell If He Fancies You

Male body language is fairly obvious, hence the infamous Mae West quote, 'Is that a pistol in your pocket or are you just pleased to see me?' Well, you may not see an erection but look out for the following when you clap eyes on him:

The double take He spots you, looks away but can't resist going back for a second look quite quickly. This is a dead give away – unless you've got a massive spot on your nose that he can't take his eyes off!

He only has eyes for you Even if a gorgeous girl walks past he barely notices. His glances keep going in your direction.

His posture He pulls himself up so he's standing straight and he may link his fingers into his belt loop in a subconscious gesture to draw your eyes to his manhood.

He smiles! A simple smile speaks volumes – he wants a smile back!

His walk He begins to saunter that masculine walk.

The chat-up He gets talking to you – it may even be about something inane – so talk back. Ask him a question to keep the conversation flowing.

The bridge He touches your forearm as he speaks to you, bringing your personal spaces together.

The block He moves so that his upper body is blocking you from the rest of the bar/nightclub/whatever – literally blocking off any competition from clapping eyes on you.

'Check me out' He keeps looking over at the lads for approval to say 'check out my success'. He really fancies you – or his chances!

Sexual Confidence — Know Thyself

The first step to sexual confidence is finding out how your body works. This is crucial. There should be no shame in exploring your own sexual responses through masturbation. One research survey found 98 per cent of men said they had masturbated, while only 75 per cent of women said they had. Some were fibbing, of course, but sadly too many women I come across have a fear of touching or looking at their own body – even in our modern times.

'Mirror, mirror' Get a mirror, lie back and simply look at your genitals. Examine every little inch of your vagina, labia, clitoris, anus and perineum (the area between the vulva and the anus). The more you look the more comfortable you'll feel.

Tender touch Ensure you're comfortable. If you haven't masturbated before, start by caressing your breasts, arms, abdomen and thighs – anywhere you can reach that feels good! You can do this sitting or lying comfortably, or in the bath or shower. Use some massage oil or lubricant to heighten sensations. If you really have a problem about touching your genitals, you may first want to touch yourself through your knickers to build confidence. Caress yourself slowly. Enjoy the sensations. Build to fully touching yourself as your excitement increases. This is a good, healthy thing to do. It's not 'dirty' or 'sordid' – so don't let anyone tell you that!

Keep this in mind. Women are NOT mind readers, and men are even worse! How can your lover guess how to pleasure you if you won't even learn about your own responses?

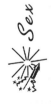

Sexual Confidence II – Building To Orgasm

The female orgasm – or climax – is complicated. Only about 20 per cent of women regularly climax through penetrative sex with their partners. Most need to use a combination of stimulation – hands, oral sex, sex toys, and so on, to help them on their way during sex. Depending on the study, some 15 per cent or so of women never climax during penetrative sex.

So, by learning how to bring yourself to orgasm through masturbation, you can then put this knowledge to good use with a lover – and recreate the sensations you know work for you. This means lots of experimenting when you're not in a rush. Now that you've experienced pleasurable sensations during masturbation it may still take you some exploring to find out how to get all the way to orgasm.

Feel free to try different things. For example, some women find they can only climax by using the palm of their hand, or by rubbing against a pillow or cushion. Others like to introduce a vibrator or dildo (a penis-shaped sex toy that doesn't vibrate) to help them on their way. This is where Frank Sinatra comes in handy – live by his saying, 'I did it my way' and you can't go wrong!

Some women experience orgasm as a slow build-up of sexual tension with a powerful release that may come in waves. Others experience a quick build-up with a short release. Still others feel a much more gentle form of sensual experience. On average, an orgasm lasts about 6–8 seconds. Hold in mind what works for you – for example, vigorous finger stimulation or a gentle rubbing – to teach your lover.

Sexual Confidence III – You're A Love And Sex Goddess

Visualisations work! Cancer patients who visualise strong white blood cells cleaning up their systems have been found to have an increased production of these important cells. Those who visualise for academic work can achieve scores 10 per cent higher. And footballers who visualise their last great goal are more likely to score another. It's all about gaining a positive mindset. So *you* can visualise being a love goddess!

Get comfortable *in* something really sexy – feeling that you *look* sexy will help you visualise yourself as a sex goddess. Recline in a big armchair or easy chair where you're warm enough in your slinky little negligée. Close your eyes and take a few relaxing breaths. Feel your breasts move up and down gently with your breathing. Allow your legs to relax and your hands to flop by your sides, unless you wish to touch yourself.

Now visualise someone you think of as being really sexy – maybe an icon like Marilyn Monroe, or someone in the news right now. Run your eyes over her image. What makes her sexy and sensuous? What are her qualities? Maybe she's just gorgeous and voluptuous. Maybe she's got real character. What you think counts.

Now imagine yourself having those qualities – you lolling about loving every inch of your sensual self. Place this image on a pedestal surrounded by sex slaves pandering to your every whim. You are this gorgeous amazing sex goddess. Affirm to yourself that you are *worthy* of great sex. Hold this image each day for a few moments.

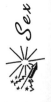

A Big Secret To Boost Your Confidence Further

He's as worried as you are! He's cute, he's in between your sheets and you're having a panic attack in your loo thinking you're going to let him down in bed – your sexual confidence has plummeted to a big fat zero! Well guess what – that hunk warming your sheets is just as worried about having sex with you! Having chatted to thousands of men in my role as agony aunt and life coach, 99.9 per cent worry about the first time they sleep with you. 'Will I be too fast?' 'Will I lose my erection?' (two of the most common male sexual fears) And, 'Will her ex-lovers be better then me?' So relax – you both may be a bundle of nerves – this is human. Taking it slowly will help you feel (literally!) your way through your first lovemaking session. It's not a competition to see who's more experienced. It's about getting to know each other.

So how do you do this? You undress each other slowly – unless it's one of those hot *just-in-the-door-rip-each-other's-clothes-off-and-do-it-standing-up* jobs! And that means you're both sexually confident. Take time lingering over his buttons or zips. Build this into foreplay. Make his heart skip a few beats by allowing this time to build up.

Give him the confidence to take his time with you, too. Whisper that you're not in a rush and you want to take it slowly. Sometimes women have to take charge of building this sort of confidence. Go for it – you'll both have a better time leading to increased sexual confidence!

Developing Your Sex Muscles

You can greatly enhance your sex life and genital health by exercising your sex muscles – the pubococcygeal (PC, or 'pelvic floor') muscles. Research has found that the strength and tone of these muscles contribute to sexual pleasure and orgasmic capability in women. And in men, exercising PC muscles can contribute greatly to learning how to control their ejaculatory response – that is, they can last longer. How do you identify your PC muscles? Think about when you're spending a penny and you want to stop the flow of urination. These are the muscles that allow you to do that. The best way to exercise them is to start at a low level and build slowly.

Begin with ten repetitions, twice a day. To begin with, you may wish to get comfortable sitting, lying, or standing. But once you've mastered this you'll find you can do your exercises at your desk, on the bus, anywhere. Even during sex – your lover will love the pulsing sensation as you clamp and unclamp your PC muscles. A repetition consists of tightening and holding for a count of two or three. As you gain control of your PC muscles you can build to twenty repetitions three times a day. After doing your repetitions, stroke your PC muscles and the surrounding area to relax them, running your strokes from either side of your clitoris, down the sides of your labia, to your perineum.

The benefits of a strong pelvic floor include better orgasms as well as prevention of bladder weakness (or improvement if you already have the problem). This is particularly important after pregnancy.

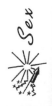

Developing Your Sex Muscles — Level II

Build your vaginal muscle strength by other inventive means. Ever thought of weight training with your vagina? You can – by using weights attached to a love 'egg' or ball. These weights can be put in a cloth bag and strung on to the little safety 'pull string' that love 'eggs' have. Or purchase solid 'eggs' on the Internet with an 'eye' to string the weights through.

Stage one simply involves working the inner vaginal muscles to hold the 'egg' in place. Start with a larger 'egg' and work down to smaller ones – this is even harder as you have to 'hang on' to them! Remember to clean any 'eggs' purchased thoroughly by disinfecting and then boiling. Next, use small weights (beware of any hooks!) bagged and attached to the 'egg'. Start with 6–9 oz (175–250 g) and ensure you don't overuse your inner muscles. Slowly build up the weight you use.

Instead of 'eggs', try *standing* and gripping a vibrator (when it's turned off, obviously!), if you've got one, as it's a harder shape to hold on to than an 'egg'. Next, begin to crouch slowly and see how far you can crouch before your muscles let the vibrator slip.

Finally, why not go for a bit of a flutter. Once your pelvic floor muscles are stronger you'll find that not only can you contract and release them anywhere, any time, but you can flutter them. Imagine the way a belly dancer rolls her stomach – try this with your pelvic floor.

The Best Sex

You can settle for OK sex but I hope you want more. I'm not talking now about technique and choosing crazy sexual positions or the weirdest stuff you can do without being classed as a raving pervert. I'm talking about simply enjoying sex on *your* terms. Having chatted to thousands of women, there seem to be two criteria for deciding how much good or bad sex they're getting. These are: when they wait long enough (*see* 'One-Night Stands' in Part Two: 'Guys – Love', page 60) to feel they can *communicate* with their lover, and when they feel in *control.*

***Communication* first** Think about this – if you're only just getting to know a man and wouldn't feel comfortable discussing your mother's alcoholism, your uncle's depression, or a recent humiliation at work – how on earth can you discuss sex and likes/dislikes/fantasies/and so on? If you can't discuss it, how will it be safer and enjoyable? Too many women close their eyes (not literally but metaphorically!) hoping for the best – not daring to say anything to a new lover about sex. Not good! If you wait until you can talk about it before having sex it'll be better sex – I guarantee it.

Next there's *control* You'll have far better sex if you're in control. By control I mean – when you want it, in a place you want it, and how you want it. The simple rule? Don't have it *until you want it.* you know you're going to enjoy it as you're not sneaking behind parents' or flatmates' backs, and you feel absolutely ready.

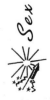

Before-play

Before-play is a concept I first introduced into sex advice about five years ago. After speaking to vast numbers of women – especially those who'd lost desire – I realised that there wasn't enough good stuff going on *before* sex to put them in the mood to even start. So I coined the term 'before-play' to remind people of the importance of how you feel *generally* in your life and about the man in your life, and the effect this has on how sexy you feel. This is just as important with a new lover as one you've been with for a long time.

I talk about general principles of emotional well-being and fitness in Part Three: 'Chocolate – Life', so I'll stick with issues of romance here. If you two have loads of stress in your life, or are edgy being in a new relationship with each other (maybe due to past 'baggage'), or have just argued – you won't be in the mood for sex (although some couples adore make-up sex!). So never forget the principles of romance, respect and generally having loads of goodwill for each other and the role it plays in making you feel sexy.

If, for example, your long-term lover has just forgotten your birthday, or your new man is more interested in himself than you, then you will not feel very sexy. He'll feel the same way if you neglect him. Before the first hint of foreplay begins, make romantic gestures, be affectionate, see the good in each other and generally care for each other – and sex will stay alive for you!

Getting What You Want

The women who get what they want in bed have the sexual confidence to communicate and take control, and are also good at the *give and take* of great sex. Let's begin with *'taking'* first – more fun! There are many ways of getting a man to pleasure you. These are the most effective:

✓ Men love to be asked! Use a sexy and seductive voice and *ask* him for what you want. If you preface this by saying, *'I know you'll be so good at it* so will you please dribble this massage oil over my buttocks and swirl it around?' you'll have him on his knees dying to do it for you!

✓ Show him how to do it! For example, if you love your nipples being sucked in a particular way, then suck his in that way, look up at him with a naughty smile and say, 'Will you suck my nipples like that, too?' Or, take his finger (or even his penis!) and suck it with the pressure and style you love and say, 'It'd feel fantastic if you sucked my nipples like this!'

✓ Use pictures! Take his favourite men's mag – or your girl's mag – or a sex guide like my book *Sinful Sex – The Uninhibited Guide to Erotic Pleasure*, and show him a photo, article or passage that describes what you'd like to do.

✓ Move him into position! You can always take his hand, his head (!), his penis, and so on, and move it to where you want it, creating the action that turns you on.

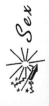

Giving Him What He Wants

Just as it's rewarding for you to get good 'technique' given to you – so it's rewarding to give him what he wants. Loads of women think it's 'tarty' to be too good in bed – utter rubbish! You'll both be happier if you know that your lover's satisfied. Try these most effective methods:

✓ Ask him what he wants! You'll not be seen as a scarlet woman if you whisper, 'What would you like me to do?' as you run your fingers down his chest. No, he'll see you as a Sex Goddess straight from heaven and will eagerly tell you his likes.

✓ Experiment and listen to his sex noises! Try different techniques and simply listen to his responses. Unless he's 'Mr Silent-type', men let slip little noises that tell you whether or not you're hitting the spot. So stay tuned to his sex sounds.

✓ Describe a sex scene to him! Telling him about something you think he'll like can have two effects: *1* you'll hit it on the button and it's something he likes too, or *2* you'll introduce him to something new. So if you love the 'feeding frenzy' between Mickey Rourke and Kim Bassinger in *9½ Weeks* say, 'It'd be fantastic to drip cream down your chest and between your thighs to lick off gently!'

✓ Map out his erogenous zones! Tell him you're on a mission of discovery. With a feather, basting brush, end of a whip – trace all around his body, asking what feels best – and remember his answers!

Feeling Sexy — Your Timing And His

Depending on your own sexual 'clock' you may feel horniest during ovulation (when your body says it's time to make babies), or just before your period, owing to hormonal changes, or, for some women, after their period, when they feel calm and in control. Men also peak at different times as their testosterone levels change – often over a 24-hour period. Some are morning-men – others are naughty at night.

When sleeping with each other for the first time, you may both feel like sex all the time. But it's quite natural for things to settle down after three to six months. At this point, your essential levels of sex drive may determine whether or not you experience problems in this department. Many couples find that one or the other 'feels like it' more frequently than the other. You *can* sort this out.

First, when the first flush of lust starts to dwindle, neither of you should take it personally – talk about it. Second, it's critical to keep the romance going (so neither of you feels neglected) as well as building in a few new sex tricks to keep things lively *when you do have sex*. Next, take turns initiating sex so you both feel you're keeping things alive. It's easy for the one with a higher sex drive to do all the initiating – this can get annoying. Finally, if there are big differences in your sex drives, ask: is sex being used to play out other difficulties? Is one of you over-worked, stressed or ill?

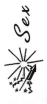

Blissful Kissing

Your lips are so packed with nerve endings, research shows that even a gentle brush across them can stimulate an area in the brain larger than the one stimulated by a touch to your genitals! Your lips also swell slightly and deepen in colour when you're attracted to someone or sexually aroused. Kissing is incredibly intimate, which is why many prostitutes will do everything *but!*

The first kiss: if you'd like to kiss him but aren't sure if he wants to, simply move in closer, ensure your head is tilted up to his and speak in soft tones. This'll increase his kissing confidence. Many women (and men!) worry about how to kiss a man. Here are some tips for a sensational snog:

1   Practise on the *inside* of your wrist to gauge what your lips feel like when in kissing mode.
2   Check out your oral hygiene – is your breath fresh?
3   Loosen your lips as you go in for the kill. Tight lips are a turn-off!
4   Allow your tongue to relax too – only use it in a stiff poking kiss with the suggestions below. Let it swirl around the inside of his lips and the roof of his mouth (both neglected places that feel great when gently stimulated) as well as circling his tongue with yours.
5   Just go with the moment – it may be a gentle or passionate kiss but people who fancy each other have a subconscious way of getting there in the end – even if their noses bump at first!

Advanced Kissing

A few advanced kissing techniques can turn you into a great lover. Here are some favourites to try.

The Medieval Necklet Encircle the delicate skin on your lover's neck with little kisses. Start behind his ear and plant wet little kisses, making a circle that goes down his collar bone, ending up behind his other ear.

The Vacuum Allow your lips to relax then encircle your lover's closed lips. Gently apply a little sucking – or vacuum – to his outer lips and pulsate slowly. You are in control. The delicate skin around his lips will be stimulated and feel fantastic.

The Snake As the name suggests, you ease your tongue across your lover's lips, into his mouth and *anywhere* on his body in little flicking motions. Great for flicking little crumbs of food off his body after food-play.

These are techniques to ask your lover to try on you:

The Naughty Dog This passionate, earthy kiss is great for larger erogenous zones like the whole breast, abdomen and inner thigh. Ask your lover to start at the base of your breast and lap upwards, flicking your nipple as he finishes the lap. He can use it on the inner thigh, finishing the lap with a gentle flick, going down your inner thigh towards the knee or up towards the genitals.

The Eastern Swirl and Poke Originating in the Far East, this feels heavenly. Ask your lover to use it with a French kiss or on your body. He first swirls around with his tongue encircling yours, then pokes gently with the tip of his tongue. This feels great on the nipples, around the tummy button and genitals.

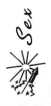

Sex

Oral Sex — Getting Started

Oral sex is a deeply intimate act that can give enormous pleasure, but it can also create great anxiety. Men and women worry about giving *and receiving* oral sex. Their concerns usually involve fear about how to do it and personal hygiene – will *they* like the taste of their lover – or will their lover like the way *they* taste?

Hygiene Good hygiene's essential for you both. A bit of water play (*see page 36*) can get you both *fresh* in a sensual way. But if it's not convenient to have a bath/shower together, wash on your own before lovemaking, or introduce a warm, wet face cloth to carefully wash each other as part of foreplay. Don't forget that many women are sensitive to commercial douches/soaps/shower gels, which, ironically, can lead to irritation and a smell.

Safer oral You can transfer nasty bugs between the mouth and the genitals. Herpes Simplex I of the mouth can be passed to the genitals and Herpes Simplex II can be carried from the genitals to the mouth. If you don't know his sexual history, use flavoured condoms and give him a blow job through them. He should cover you with a dental dam/cling film and give you 'head' through that.

Get your tongue ready Your tongue/lips should be in shape to give all sorts of sensations. Each day, flick your tongue up and down to build its strength. Then circle it round and round. Practise swirling your lips around one of your fingers so you know what it'll feel like on the tip of his glans.

Oral Sex II – Getting It From Him

Tongue techniques There are all sorts of tongue techniques he can use on you. Ask him to kiss, flick and lick down your abdomen, across your mons pubis, down either side of your labia and your inner thighs. Not coming into contact with your clitoris will leave you panting for more.

Nose and lips If you have a sensitive clitoris, ask him to use his lips and nose (yes!) to gently stimulate you. Ask him *not* to draw back your clitoral hood, too. By placing your hands behind his ears you can control the pressure he uses.

Loving the pearl When you're aroused, guide him to put his thumb and forefinger on either side of your clitoris and *gently* rub it – lots of lubricant will make this heavenly!

V for victory If you don't like clitoral stimulation, this is an alternative way to make you climax. He makes a 'V' sign and slips his two fingers, palm down, on either side of your clit, pointing down your labia. He can then gently circle his 'V' sign, arousing all the nerve endings around your mons pubis, clitoris and labia.

Finger work Take his fingers and place them where you want, to show him the pressure you like near your clitoris. He can 'drum' lightly, rub in circular motions, twirl your labia or around the clitoral region to give you wonderful sensations.

Come on over Perfect for him to stimulate your G-spot while sucking your labia or clitoris. With palm upwards, ask him to insert his index and middle fingers inside your vagina. Then he does a gentle 'come here' gesture – repeatedly.

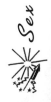

Oral Sex III — Giving It To Him

Mouth Magic You can lap, suck, flick and tease with your tongue and lips. Ask how the different sensations feel! Practise on a penis-shaped vibrator (switched off!) to build your confidence. Get him to 'direct' you.

Swirling Perfect for around the penile glans, swirling is sensual and loving. Ensure your tongue stays loose as, with a leisurely pace, you swirl lightly. You may wish to increase the pressure of your tongue as his arousal increases.

Snaking Hold your tongue loosely and allow it to slip sideways back and forth quite quickly. This feels amazing early in oral play with its gentle sweeping sensation. Start at the lower abdomen, then move down to his genitals.

Funnelling Imagine you're savouring a Polo mint. Holding the imaginary Polo in front of your mouth, you curl your tongue like a funnel, slipping it in and out of the hole in the centre. Funnelling can be used on men who like the opening of their urethra stimulated.

Humming While holding either his glans or a testicle in your mouth hum gently – he'll love the vibes!

Hand and mouth Use your hands, too. If your mouth tires, switch to using both hands – one at the base of his penis, one at the tip. Move them in and out first towards, and then away from, each other.

Deep throat Many women never get past the gag reflex. Your throat should be lined up straight with your jaw (head back) propped by pillows.

And finally If you hate giving 'head' kiss *around* his genitals. Or spread your favourite topping (jam, chocolate) over him and eat it off. Don't be pressured into any sex act you dislike!

Touch

Most people don't realise how many different sensations they can give and receive by simply changing the way they touch. Even changing from touching your lover with your right hand, to using your left hand will vary the sensations.

Try bringing the scalp alive with a few gentle touches to the earlobe, then circling behind the neck as you two kiss. As you touch your lover, listen to his love sounds – be guided. If he loves something, don't feel you have to move on. We're all in such a rush for the genitals! Don't be! Linger over what feels good to him. A big rule to remember – at different times you'll both want different areas touched. Spoil each other by taking turns touching different parts. One of you lies back while the other tickles, teases, scratches, and swirls their fingers over the other's body.

Other things to try Trickle some lubricant down his stomach and swirl a feather through it. For a firmer touch, drag a clean kitchen basting brush through the lube. Why not wear some soft gloves or latex ones with lots of lube to stimulate each other? Run a vibrator over his well-lubricated skin. Keep your nails clean and short, unless he loves a scratching sensation. Check this out – some men hate being scratched!

Don't forget Inside the wrists, behind the knees, across the ankles, stroking individual toes, massaging the hands, caressing around and down the ribs. Swish your fingers back and forth, up and down the inner thighs and buttocks.

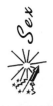

New Sexual Thrills – Developing Your Sexth Sense!

Listen to your lover. He may drop hints. Sometimes one of you might suggest something the other's turned off by – like anal sex. This doesn't mean one of you is a 'perve' and the other a prude – no judgements please, or you'll both be wary of suggesting new things.

Balloons The challenge here is for him to thrust while keeping the balloons between you – without popping them.

Jet stream Using a balloon, control a thin stream of air across your lover's lubed-up body – this feels fantastic on the genitals.

Ice and wax play Alternate sensations – first trail ice over his skin with your fingers or between your lips. Then drop a little melted wax from *one metre* – testing first on the inside of your wrist. WARNING – You or your lover can get burnt if you're not careful! You're responsible for testing the wax! Or dribble warm water over the spot you've just iced. Ensure the water is a comfortable temperature.

Stripping Take turns stripping for each other. Practise on your own, then turn down the lights, put on some mood music and bump and grind slowly. You'll either get very turned on or laugh – both are good!

Al fresco *and other places* Be careful of outdoors sex in your back garden if it is overlooked. Make *al fresco* sex as risky and fun as you want. Find a truly deserted beauty spot, or slip out of a party into the toilet to have a quickie!

Spanking and whipping Start gently and move across his flesh – you don't want bruising – or do you!? Try a satin sash or cloth belt before moving up to leather.

Sex Positions

Guess what? Research shows couples stick to two or three favourites – because it's easy. But down the line it gets boring, such as sticking to 'spoons' on Friday night. A few worth trying:

Spoons Lying side by side, he penetrates from behind.

Doggy He is behind while she is on all fours, facing down.

The spinner He's on his back, she sits astride him and eases around first 90 degrees, so that she's sides on, then 180 degrees so that her back's to him. She controls thrusting. If he's a 'bum man' he'll love the view.

The double header He can push himself up from *the spinner* and they continue with her back pressed into his chest. Or he sits back against the sofa or bed-head and she slips on to his lap with her back to his chest. A gentle 'ride'.

The sling Standing with him supported by a wall, facing each other, she moves a leg up over his arm, so that it forms a 'sling', and gives better access for penetrating her.

The ploughman She's on her back, legs up, knees bent into his chest. He balances on his feet while crouching and holds her buttocks, bringing them to meet his thrusts. He can lean his hands into the bed or floor (or wherever they are!).

The puppet He stands behind her. She bends forward like a limp puppet and either rests her hands on a bed or sofa, or, if flexible, on the floor. This gives him great G-spot access. Don't forget the 'U' and 'A' spots. The 'U' is located just below the clitoris and above the urethral opening. The 'A' (*anterior fornix*) is deeper in the vagina, past the 'G'.

31

Sex Toys

Lovers should use sex toys together more often. They're fun, feel good and add to your lovemaking in many ways. And even though many women use vibrators they often hide this fact from the men in their lives. For hygiene, keep separate 'his' and 'her' bags of sex toys and clean them as instructed.

Men love the idea of playing with toys – but they're also a bit shy about admitting this. So start with something non-threatening, such as a small vibrator. If you thrust one of those huge vibrators in his face he'll *a* be very ashamed of his penis size and *b* find the device hard to handle! Some great toys on the market include:

Penis-shaped vibrator Have fun vibrating up and down your nipples, abdomen, perineum – and his!

Jessica Rabbit or *Pearl Rabbit vibrator* These have 'ears' to stimulate the clitoris during penetration with the vibrator.

G-spot, *clit-tickler*, *fingertip* and *bullet-style vibrators* These are usually designed as flexible wands with vibrating ends to hit the spot.

Anal vibrators/butt plugs For those of you willing to try something new.

Tongue Joy A mini-vibrator that slips on your lover's tongue to give you joy everywhere he kisses you!

Vibrating cushion He sits on it – she sits astride him and during penetration the vibrations come up between them.

Penile shaft sleeves A huge variety of soft and flexible sleeves can be worn on finger or penis. They have bumps for extra stimulation. Check out www.blushingbuyer.co.uk

Sexy Feasts and Aphrodisiacs

Sliding between the sheets with a few pieces of chocolate, to warm up and smooth over erogenous zones, or enjoying a whole sexy feast in bed, is incredibly sensual. We forget that our mouths are centres of eroticism – be creative! Slip morsels of food into your lover's mouth. Hold a ripe strawberry dipped in cream between your lips and share. Here are some fabulous foods/additives that seem sexy and may have aphrodisiac properties:

Almonds These contain properties said to revive flagging desire. Mediterranean cultures bake them into savouries and desserts as love-symbols.

Asparagus Hand-feed your lover warm spears dripping with melted butter.

Bananas These give energy and contain alkaloids with aphrodisiac effects. Bake with sugar and spices, and spoon-feed your lover.

Chocolate This contains phenyl-ethylamine and caffeine, which stimulate the brain, and sugar, which boosts energy.

Ginger, cinnamon and ginseng powders The Chinese have used ginger as a stimulant for 3,000 years. Eastern cultures use cinnamon and ginseng for the same purpose – bake or sprinkle on to food.

Oysters and other seafood These contain zinc, which is beneficial for energy levels – and they look so sexy!

Avena sativa Buy in extract form and add to food and drinks. This seems to help those with low testosterone.

Damania A popular aphrodisiac grown in hot climates and purchased in capsule or tincture forms, it contains alkaloids that boost circulation.

Gingko biloba Known to increase blood and oxygen flow.

Muira puama Popular in Germany – this can be brewed or taken as a capsule.

Yohimbine This may increase male libido, possibly by boosting neurotransmitters.

WARNING Don't take any supplements without consulting your doctor first.

Sexual Fantasies

About 95 per cent of men and 75 per cent of women own up to having some sort of sexual fantasy life. I actually think it's about 98 per cent ACROSS THE BOARD! Only a few people are so sexually inhibited or uninterested that their minds don't wander into sexual territory from time to time. Many women are simply embarrassed to admit to having them. Why? Because women still worry it makes them seem 'slutty'. This is ridiculous. Having sexual fantasies is great!

Relish these quiet moments as they may prove to be a fertile ground for spicing up your sex life. The human mind is constantly asking, 'What if?' We wouldn't have evolved to the supposedly 'civilised' people we are if our minds weren't always dreaming up new things to try. So, when it comes to sexual *'What ifs?'* – such as, 'What if my boss threw me across the photocopier and ravished me?, 'What if my neighbour caught me in the nude?' or 'What if that sexy doctor gave me an intimate examination?' – they can generate all sorts of shared fantasies and role plays. Top female fantasises include power themes – dominating a man, being powerless, sex with strangers, and lesbian sex.

Believe it or not, men find it terribly exciting to fantasise about what *you might be fantasising* about! Men seem to think we're so complicated when many of our fantasises are as earthy and basic as theirs. The important thing to remember is how to let them in on your naughty little fantasy life . . . coming next!

Etiquette For Sharing Your Fantasies And Other Desires

Here are half a dozen rules for sharing your fantasies:

1   Always introduce your fantasy life gently – don't storm in with, 'I only get turned on thinking about having a three-some!' So, for example, if 'three-way' is your fantasy, start with, 'Have you ever wondered what it'd be like to have a threesome?'

2   Always clarify that this is fantasy time – not something you want to make into a reality! Do not be pressured by a partner into turning fantasy chat into a reality.

3   Always praise your partner first – this is something that'll come up repeatedly in smoothing the path of your relationships. Think of something your lover does that genuinely turns you on. For example, say, 'I love it when you stroke the backs of my thighs and buttocks, it makes me imagine that I'm lying down, sunbathing on a beach and you don't know me and you walk up and start rubbing suntan lotion into my back, buttocks, and legs . . .'. Then you've built a compliment straight into a fantasy.

4   If it turns out that your particular fantasy kink is a real turn-off for your lover, find another one that won't make him feel uneasy. Feeling pressured to share a fantasy can actually end up ruining your sex life.

5   Once you are both confident enough to chat about your fantasy lives, build in some role play. For example, if you're both turned on by a 'stranger sex' fantasy, then meet up in a bar as 'strangers in the night' and get carried away.

6   The power of fantasy can't be underestimated. When you are comfortable sharing these desires it'll liven things up – and that's what we want!

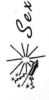

Water Play

Water is sexy – gushing, surging, splashing – it frees you up! But many women feel a little uncomfortable about what could happen during water play – how will we actually *shag*? You don't have to go the 'full monty' if your bath or shower is small. But you can still have fun.

Start by using candles to light your bath or shower room so that it looks really seductive. Turn on some mood music. You could start water play by leading your partner into the bath and simply offer to wash him or give him a back massage. This way you can slowly get into the mood to try other things. Use the showerhead to spray him (and he you) gently from neck to toes. But don't let him spray the shower directly up into your vagina as, in *rare* circumstances, you may blast an air bubble into the bloodstream.

Lather each other up with a bath or shower gel that neither of you reacts to (don't forget your genitals may get irritated when using some products). Take turns simply washing each other's shoulders and breasts with loads of lather. Introduce one of the new waterproof sex toys to your water play – water plus vibrations feels fab! The 'water duck' is definitely good fun. Beware – you can't use condoms in the bath or shower. So, if you want to use a condom, gently towel each other down – this can be incredibly sensual with big warm, fluffy towels – and then head for the bedroom.

Finally, rub loads of moisturiser or lube slowly into each other's skin. A sensual massage finishes off water play perfectly.

All Tied Up

Many people find the idea of some 'vanilla' bondage a real turn on. 'Vanilla' means a gentle, fairly straight, non-threatening sort of sexual activity. There are seven points to consider when thinking about introducing a little bondage play into your sex life:

1 Talk about it first. Maybe while changing your clothes, you can ask your lover to let you tie his tie. Use this opportunity to say, 'Wow, it'd be cool if we put this tie to another use – like on your wrists or mine!'

2 If he seems agreeable and not shocked, next time you make love have a tie handy by the bedside, or wherever you are. Or, if your lover doesn't wear ties, then a dressing gown sash.

3 Always tie with 'bows' not knots – I can't tell you how many novices have got themselves all tied up in knots and it's taken the pleasure out of the 'event'.

4 Tie loosely enough to ensure that your lover doesn't feel threatened.

5 Agree a word that actually means you want to 'stop'. In the heat of the moment you may say something like, 'Stop! Stop!' as part of the fantasy play, so choose a neutral word, then your lover knows you're serious.

6 Never leave anyone tied up. Don't tie each other up if you've been drinking excessively or taking drugs.

7 Build up a bedside bondage bag of goodies. Things like handcuffs, different restraints, or blindfolds. Get some bondage sheets with Velcro wrist/ankle straps!

Check out www.fetteredpleasures.com

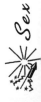

Your Sex Treasure Chest

A big complaint I hear from women is that there's never anything new in their lovemaking. It's – get into position, do it, and roll over. If you want to make your sex life more spontaneous you have to do some planning. That way, when you two are feeling randy, you've got a selection of playthings to suit your mood. Stock up a lockable (if you have children) chest by the bed for all your goodies. This should include:

✓ Lubricants and massage oils. If using condoms, only use water-based lubricants or those specifically safe for condoms. Also, don't allow oils to get inside the vagina – they can irritate your delicate pH balance.

✓ Your favourite sex toys, such as handcuffs, vibrators, and 'clit' ticklers. Store them in 'his' and 'hers' bags to keep them extra hygienic.

✓ A soft, satiny blindfold and sexy dice for sex games.

✓ Your favourite erotica to read to each other, or erotic films to watch together.

✓ Soft ties or stockings for bondage play and dressing up.

✓ A feather or basting brush for touching techniques.

✓ Condoms, dental dams, cling film and latex gloves for safer sex play – if you don't know your partner's sexual history.

✓ Erotic edibles – chocolates and honey don't need refrigeration and are perfect for sex play.

✓ Your favourite mood music CD so it's not lost among the rest of your music collection when the time is right.

✓ A box of luxury tissues – need I say more?

Check out www.Myla.com

Forbidden Practices –
Anal Sex For Him And Her

Anal sex has been practised by various cultures throughout history. The enlightened Sumerians practised hetero- and homosexual anal sex. Often anal sex was used to give pleasure without fear of pregnancy. That said, many still have a taboo about such 'forbidden' practices. Explore this tactfully with your lover. No one should feel pressured into anal sex who's put off by it. However, anal sex is not advisable unless you know your partner's sexual history as there is an increased risk of HIV transmission. Always use a condom, avoiding those that contain the spermicide N-9.

➤ The rectum needs to be emptied, naturally or with a suppository.
➤ Expel any wind first – going to the bathroom, getting on all fours and tilting your bottom upwards helps! This'll prevent some embarrassing noises.
➤ Ensure your anal area and hands are clean.
➤ Relaxation is incredibly important. Tension means the outer sphincter won't relax, causing pain. Foreplay should help with arousal and relaxation of the anal area.
➤ Use loads of water-based lubricant. Unlike the vagina, the anal passage is not naturally lubricated. Re-apply generously!
➤ Try simple touching and then gentle partial finger penetration (wearing latex gloves) to stimulate this delicate area. Trim your nails for finger play!
➤ To get started, try inserting one latex-gloved finger into the anus. Keep it still, allowing the sphincter to relax.
➤ Build to penetration with the penis, anal vibrator, or strap-on – for the man who wants to be penetrated! The person being penetrated should control the depth and speed of thrusting.
➤ Individuals have different tastes in terms of positions. Some prefer 'spoons', others 'doggy' and others the 'double header' (see page 31).

Sex

When He's Too Quick

Men have complicated feelings about sex. Yes, when it suits them (one-night stands!) they can switch off emotionally and totally enjoy a physical moment. But their sense of worth is bound up in their performance. Many dread one of two problems: coming too quickly – premature ejaculation (PE) – and losing their erection (*next page*). Men frequently experience PE out of sheer excitement, especially when having 'first-time' sex with someone new (90 per cent of men have reported this happening with at least one partner). Other men get into a habit of PE (often learned as a teen when they rushed for fear of discovery) that they find hard to break. These six steps will help a man who is experiencing PE:

1   Encourage him to build his PC muscle (*see page 17*) then . . .
2   Through masturbation, he identifies his 'point of no return' – where he *has* to ejaculate. Before this point is the plateau stage. This is where developing stronger PC muscles helps. As he reaches his 'point', some simple squeezes of the PC muscles will help him to stop ejaculating.
3   He should introduce this new control gradually into love-making.
4   During lovemaking, he can concentrate on your sensations first – building his confidence.
5   Use positions that give less friction during penetration. This'll also help him control his PE. In these positions he can stimulate you with his hand or a sex toy.
6   For some men, 'second time around' is much slower and, as well as practising the above, he may be happy to have second, slower go!

When His Erection Fails

One in ten men experience erectile dysfunction (ED) at some point in their life. Over 2,300,000 men experience this in Britain alone. Usually it is transitory but it rocks a man's confidence to the core if it happens. It may occur in response to a heavy drinking session or drug taking or as a side-effect of medicine or a physical disorder, such as diabetes. It can also be emotional.

If he can get and maintain an erection during masturbation, or if he wakes with a morning erection, then the problem is likely to be emotional. For example, he feels threatened in the relation-ship, or it is in response to a lifestyle choice – perhaps he drinks heavily at night and then can't 'get it up'.

Encourage your partner to masturbate and experiment privately with his erection. This can build his confidence and openness between you. If he can't get an erection, or only has a partial erection – even when *on his own* – he needs to look at physical causes. He should book a double appointment with his doctor. If he has a woman doctor and feels embarrassed, he may request a male doctor. A double appointment will allow for more time to explore what can be a sensitive issue. Please remember – doctors have heard this problem a thousand times. If he's not happy with his doctor's response he should go to another one. There's no reason why he shouldn't get good advice. Also, visit www.informED.co.uk. In the meantime, you two should engage in affectionate/sensual touching and discuss whether he should simply pleasure you. You should not try to 'make him' get an erection.

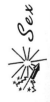

41

Women's Sexual Problems

Aside from lacking sexual confidence or not being able to talk about sex, women may experience a number of sexual difficulties. A recent study found that 43 per cent of women 'lacked sexual interest' – however, this is open to interpretation. Debate has ensued about whether the high result is down to certain issues such as lifestyle choices (for instance, overworking), psychological problems (such as depression) and relationship difficulties (constant arguing will put you off even the hottest 'make-up sex'). Many people are also sceptical about drug companies wanting to cash in on Female Sexual Dysfunction or FSD (the blanket term) by choosing to 'medicalise' it rather than looking at it holistically.

Problems that could have an emotional or physical (or combined) basis include:

Vaginismus Painful spasms of the vaginal muscles before or during intercourse.

Dyspareunia Pain before, during or after intercourse that many view as distinct from vaginismus. It can be located in different parts of the genitals and is accompanied by varying symptoms, such as vaginal dryness.

Desire problems No longer feeling sexual desire.

Female Sexual Arousal Disorder (FSAD) When a woman feels desire but can't get physically aroused for sex.

Anorgasmia or Female Orgasmic Disorder A woman's inability to achieve orgasm, even with adequate stimulation. There are a variety of causes, whether anatomical, medical, emotional or concerning relationships.

Testosterone Low levels of testosterone or other hormonal imbalances can lower a woman's sex drive.

For professional advice, speak to your GP for a referral or contact the British Association for Counselling and Psychotherapy (www.bacp.co.uk) to see a sex therapist.

Lack Of Desire For Sex

There are many reasons why women end up lacking sexual desire. Up to 40 per cent of women complain of lack of desire at some point.

'*Too tired for sex*' This is a frequent complaint! I ask a woman to assess her lifestyle. Very often we find she loves her partner and essentially there's no problem in the relationship. However, she simply doesn't have time to look after herself so that she's rested enough to want sex. The choice is to prioritise your relationship, so that you're up for sex on a reasonable basis, or to carry on the way you are – and risk damaging his feelings towards you.

Hormonal changes These can affect women at different stages of life: during pregnancy and after birth, during peri-menopausal and menopausal changes, as well as during monthly cycle changes. If you think that a lack of desire may be due to hormonal changes you should take a trip to the doctor so your hormones can be checked out. If this *is* found to be the cause, your doctor will advise you of available treatments.

Unhappiness in the relationship There's nothing less sexy than having loads of arguments, giving the 'silent treatment' and having general negative feelings in a relationship. Why would you want to sleep with someone you feel you loathe? Sort out the issues causing your relationship stress and you'll find your sex drive returns.

Side-effect of medication Medications you're on, such as some anti-depressants, can affect your sex drive adversely. Check this out with your doctor and see if there are alternatives you can take.

Sex

Sex Addiction

Some debate the existence of 'sex addiction'. However, I believe that it can exist, like any other addiction. Often sufferers have multiple or cross addictions involving drink or drugs. Sometimes sex addiction seems to creep up on an individual. Women, for example, may have taken a few of life's knocks and so choose inappropriate or out-of-character sexual encounters. They then feel badly and go out and try to affirm their self-worth by finding another man so that they can feel desirable. This backfires – he doesn't call – and again they feel bad. It's a vicious circle that keeps reconfirming their lack of self-worth. Some women start to feel, 'This is all I deserve.' Other women sleep with men right from the start of the relationship, before any trust has been built, and so set a pattern for life. Some signs to look for:

❖ Do you seek thrills and risks in your sexual relationships?
❖ Do you jump from one bed to another?
❖ Do you choose 'bad boys' – men who only want one thing?
❖ Do you feel worthless, empty or dirty after sexual encounters – even when you felt excited at first?
❖ Are your sexual encounters jeopardising a relationship, friendships or work in any way?
❖ Do you go out saying you won't pick up a one-night stand but break that promise to yourself?
❖ Do you take risks with your sexual health – like 'forgetting' to use condoms and/or birth control?

If you recognise yourself in these questions, you need help. Let friends/family know you are making bad choices. Get professional help. For more information ring Sex Addicts Anonymous (020-8946-2436).

Keeping Your Passion Alive

There are many reasons why couples feel disappointed with sex – usually the culprit is that they've *taken it for granted*. Unlike a car/house that is regularly 'serviced/maintained' they treat sex as something that *should just go well* – rather than needing love, care and attention. Other factors, like psychological and mental problems, can affect your desire. If you're depressed or anxious, sexual desire will flag. Lifestyle choices such as smoking, drinking and working long hours will also have a deleterious effect. Arguing and other emotional issues mean emotions in the bedroom cool off. Medical problems and the side-effect of some medications can diminish desire. So nurture your relationship and selves and your sex life won't suffer! Here are a few other tips:

Crazy little things Never forget that the best things come in small packages – and that includes ideas. For example, try 'flashlight fun' – using a torch to explore your lover's body under the covers. Or get artistic and buy body-sculpting plaster to make rude sculptures! Have fun directing your own video porn flicks – just don't lose the tapes! Buy fun, sexy surprises – there are all sorts of sex games on the market.

Outside help See an expert if things are really bad – try Relate (0845-130-4010) which has therapists who are trained in sex problems. The British Association for Counselling and Psychotherapy (www.bacp.co.uk) also offers specially trained counsellors.

Medication Your doctor may be able to prescribe a medication to suit you or your partner, such as testosterone patches, gels or tablets, or other hormone treatments, and pills such as Uprima, Cialis, Viagra or Levitra.

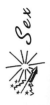

Sex

GUYS—
Love

So Do You Want A Relationship Or A Security Blanket?

The majority of women I meet say they're looking for someone *special*. They want to find a soul mate who'll make them 'feel complete'. Someone they can hold on to at night, and be there when they 'need them'. Sounds kind of like a security blanket! Men are not mystical creatures who will turn your life around, make you feel good about yourself, give you constant assurance that your bum doesn't look big (*more on that later!*), and be a lover, friend, and confidant at the same time.

This need for '*a man who . . .*' is about our relationship expectations. Where do these come from? For starters, we've all grown up on a diet of fairy tales that our 'prince' will rescue us. Second, women's magazines, and the media generally, have a lot to answer for – telling us we can expect it all from relationships. A man who can't understand and support us is not worthy of us. Can *you* understand everything about the men you date? No! Are *you* totally supportive – as well as being a complete love goddess and more? No! So this is the moment of truth, what do you expect? Be honest with yourself and write out your expectations here:

_____

_____

_____

(For example, 'I think a man should be willing to try to understand *every* part of me.' I actually had a woman say this to me in a life-coaching session recently!) Some expectations are necessary – for example, expecting a man to respect you and not cheat. Never let go of these!

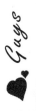

49

Your Romantic Checklist

Now for fine-tuning. Unfortunately, just as if we're shopping for groceries, women walk around with a romantic checklist in their heads detailing what a man must – and must not – have. After my divorce, my own checklist included, 'He must have children.' Why? Because I thought a man with children from a previous relationship would understand the needs of my own children. Whom did I marry? A wonderful man without children who's been an amazing stepfather. It takes a special man to do that and I met a special man.

You may not realise you've got a checklist operating in your subconscious. But you may still be guilty of ticking men *off* before they've had a chance to show their worthy qualities. Checklists put a stop to things before a man is given a chance. At different times you'll have different checklists. If you're getting broody, your checklist may include a man you can 'take to meet your parents'. If you've just come out of a long-term relationship with a control freak it may include, 'He has to be totally relaxed.' Typical things on the A to Z of romantic checklists include: he must have the 'right' sort of job. Isn't it better that he's a happy gardener than a stressed banker who puts moneymaking before you? Or 'he must be at least 5 ft 10 in'. So the most fantastic man in the world won't get a look in if he's 5 ft 8 in. If you can dare to dump your checklist, you'll meet a far wider range of men – more to choose from!

Love At First Sight

Some women believe in the love-myth that you'll know immediately if it's *'love'*. No! You'll know immediately if it's *lust*! That buzzing, exciting feeling you get when you meet someone new consists of two main things: *1* Your body chemistry has been excited by theirs. *2* Your subconscious mind has been sending and receiving all sorts of info about you to each other.

First, science has revealed how our body chemistry reacts when we meet someone we fancy. We all have special molecules known as major-histo-compatibility-complex (MHC) proteins that help the immune system identify the body's own cells. They mark us out as unique individuals. Nature knows that a couple are more likely to have a healthy baby if certain of their genes are as different as possible. And we're genetically programmed to hunt out these differences. We are helped by the fact that, almost imperceptibly, men with different MHCs *smell* different too. We subconsciously detect this faint odour and, science has shown, we prefer MHCs that are very different from our own. It's appealing to our inner 'lust' to reproduce!

Your subconscious works on the social level. What you've been used to as a child growing up – your family patterns of behaviour and relationships – you're very good at picking up when someone gives off body language you feel 'comfortable' with. That said, we make these decisions very quickly – it's a form of instant gratification. We're sent down the path of finding out more about a man by dating him because we've responded to them in the heat of those initial moments.

There's Only One True Love Out There For Me

I'm not sure where this love-myth started – maybe ancient black and white movies where the heroine, against all odds, would get her guy in the end. The message being, 'There's only one true love out there for everyone.' Let's get rid of this negative thinking – quickly!

Think about this – you probably *love* many different friends and family members. And, unless you're only just starting to date, you've probably felt *in love* with a number of men. There are loads of singles out there you could potentially share love with. The problem with believing there is 'only one' man for you is that if you've had *and lost* a past love (and maybe it left you broken hearted or finished due to circumstances at the time) you may think it'll never happen again. Many women are so hung up on the 'fact' that there can *never* be another, they cast themselves in this role. They give out the vibe that it's 'not going to happen for them' and – funnily enough – it doesn't.

We forget that men have intuition too. They're very good at reading women who are lost in 'fairy tales' – for example, that they're on a quest for the perfect man or they've loved and lost and there'll never be another. From my own experience, I know this isn't true. In the early days of my first marriage, I was deeply in love with my then husband. We had two beautiful children and I hoped we could work out our differences. I've loved since and, of course, now love my second husband. We have enormous capacity to love – so be positive!

Are You Guilty Of Problem Behaviour?

There are four general types of behaviour 'profiles' that cause problems for relationships, making them hard work and shortening their 'shelf-life'. I call these 'P'roblem behaviours or 'P' behaviours.

Prima Donna Self-centred and demanding with no empathy for others' situations – including boyfriends. You feel no one understands you. **Effect on relationships** If he doesn't worship you, you get icy and huffy. **Change** For every demand you make, give in to one of his.

People Pleaser The 'yes' person and perennial doormat who'll go along with anything. She fears standing up for herself – worries that no one will like the real her. **Effect on relationships** A man might get tired of a woman with no 'mind of her own' or he may take advantage of her willing nature. **Change** At least once daily, speak your mind. Also, choose something to do when asked, and don't say 'whatever you want'.

Passion Victim Your friends can count on you for dramatics. Unlike the Prima Donna, your dramatics revolve around their lives as much as yours. You'll make a mountain out of any molehill. **Effect on relationships** He'll find you hard work. At first curious about your dramatics, he'll tire of them over time. **Change** Calm down and enjoy letting little things roll off your back.

Perfectionist Everything must be perfect and your definition of perfect is yours. This means you're a control freak who wants things done your way. **Effect on relationships** He can never be right. You can never share doing things. He'll feel intimidated. **Change** Each day, practise doing something differently – try others' suggestions.

See 'Recognising Dysfunctional Behaviour In Ourselves' in Part Three: 'Chocolate – Life', page 115.

53

How To Put Flirting To Great Effect

Flirting makes us feel good. A recent survey found that nearly 50 per cent of men had 'flirted' in the last week, while only 37 per cent of women had. So, guys are doing it more! Research from the Social Issues Research Centre found that women use flirting to sort out their level of interest in a 'Mr Possibility'. This is why men get confused – she's flirting but then she says 'No' to a date. In Britain, and Europe generally, men use a form of 'courtesy flirting' to make a woman feel good, even though they have no intention of asking her out.

Flirting is *not* teasing! Flirting involves subtle signs of interest while teasing suggests 'action' is on the cards when it's not. Some flirting 'Dos':

✓ Giving knowing looks is a starting point – they say, 'I find you attractive.'
✓ The eyes are the windows to the soul, so ensure you've got a glint in yours.
✓ Give compliments, but only if you mean them. Men love compliments as much as we do.
✓ Be flirty with the things you say, making them sound slightly mischievous.
✓ If you've given him your number and he uses it, keep the conversation light, fun and *short* so he wants more!
✓ Be playful. During a goodnight kiss you can tickle him with your fingertips. A little flirty laughter goes a long way, too.
✓ Play obvious games. If he asks you out, say you're busy for 'two weeks' – watch his face drop and then say, 'But I can fit you in on Friday.' (Choose a day three days away.)

Where To Meet Men

Something I can't say often enough is *widen your circle of opportunity*. If you've been going to the same singles bar for three months and you haven't met anyone – go somewhere else! If you've been hanging out at the same gym and not struck lucky – choose another gym! You're responsible for choosing new venues, seizing opportunities to chat to that new man at work, and letting acquaintances know you're in the 'market'. Try speed dating, Internet sites, agencies, and the many singles events on offer in most cities. There are single men out there – no excuses!

Your safety Use these simple tips to keep safe while not inhibiting your sense of freedom and independence.

➢ Take his phone number and use '141' (to withhold your number) when dialling so that you stay in control of contact.

➢ Meet in a public place in the day time – a coffee date is always a great starting point.

➢ Tell friends or family where you're going. Or even bring a friend, particularly if you've met someone off the Internet – if he objects, it makes you wonder about his motives. Alternatively, get a friend to phone you 45 minutes into your date to check all's well, and use this call as a 'get out' if it's not going well.

➢ Keep your mobile on and carry a personal alarm – you should do this anyway.

➢ Until you know him, do not go to his home or somewhere isolated, even if you feel you trust him at first.

➢ Finally, if your intuition tells you something's wrong – believe it! We were given this 'sixth sense' to warn us of unusual body language – barely visible to the eye but clear to our subconscious.

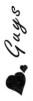

Guys

Why Men Don't Phone

You've had a couple of dates and all seems great. He's got your number now and you're anticipating date number three. But he *never* calls. You get on the phone with your friends and dissect everything. Were there any signs? Did you do something wrong? Has he had a car crash since your last date? The answer to these questions is 'No!' You haven't done anything wrong and he isn't in hospital dying. There are three main reasons why he doesn't ring:

1   Simple nerves on his part. He's wondering, 'Does she really like me?' In his little mind he decides for some reason you're not as keen as he is – so he doesn't call. He's thought of ten reasons why you might not like him. Yes, men can be that insecure – just ask a male friend.

2   You have to face facts. He decided he didn't like you enough to take it further. Most men will not do what we'd do in this situation. We'd tell a guy – 'I'm just not interested' or ' I like you as a friend'. They won't! They think it's better ('easier') to just leave things. They don't realise you're going to be tormented by insecurity.

3   Sometimes men lose the impetus. Things get in the way, particularly if he's quite independent or has lots of hobbies. He forgets to ring because he's busy. He then feels embarrassed and lets a couple of days go by. Then he decides it's too late anyway.

The message If he doesn't ring and you have his number, then ring him for a chat and sound out his enthusiasm – or lack of. If you don't have his number or he doesn't seem keen, forget him and move on!

How Men Think

Get inside a man's mind and you'd be amazed – they simply don't think the way we do. If you want to improve your relationships you need to understand this. I like to see differences as good – we complement each other. The ancient Chinese recognised this in their Yin-Yang symbolism. Difference can lead to harmony – if we *understand it* rather than treat him as an alien.

Anthropologists realise our distant ancestors had complex roles. At times, everyone in the 'cave group' had to muck in with different tasks. However, as women gave birth and suckled their offspring, their roles essentially developed around the village. They had to 'multi-task', meeting the demands of infants, the elderly, and tending any animals or plants that were raised by the group.

Men, on the other hand, had to get out in the jungle or on the plain and hunt. They had to focus on bringing down the kill and getting it home – often over long journeys, where pure survival took precedent over any niceties. They were truly goal directed, with few distractions.

How do these differences affect modern relationships? Evolution is very slow and so genetically we're still programmed to behave in these ways. Men, on the whole, like to keep things straight-forward in relationships, as in the rest of their life. They are goal directed. The goal is to get the relationship going and then let it 'tick over nicely'. Women have a strong desire to nurture things along, question the way things are, and long for deep communi-cation. A man thinks, 'The meat's on the table – what's there to talk about?'

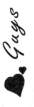

Working With The Way Men Think

To improve the relationship with your 'ancient man', you need to deal with his goal-directed thinking. Try these:

➤ We think differently – so learn from each other. Sometimes every little thing doesn't need analysis. We should take this element of men's thinking on board. When you catch yourself wanting to dissect everything about your conversation with your boss – and he's rolling his eyes – drop it. Dissect it with a girlfriend.

➤ Your type of thinking is not necessarily better than his! At the end of the day, put both thinking styles to good use. If he's got a problem with a female colleague, give him some tips to help him understand her. And vice versa.

➤ Arguments can start when either one of you refuses to acknowledge that you both may think about things differently – and they're both equally valid.

➤ It's true – two heads are better than one!

➤ Think twice before asking him what *he's thinking*. This can be incredibly annoying to a man. You're unlikely to get a straight answer. Tell him your thoughts instead, for example, 'I was thinking . . .'

➤ Don't try to read his mind. A bad habit we women have! You can't – so *ask* him, when you need to.

➤ Men's thoughts usually go from A to B. Ours go from A to K around to P and finish at Z. You don't have to share all these points with him – he'll tune you out anyway.

➤ Silence is golden. Men are often quite content with a bit of silence. It's not always negative!

How Men Feel

A typical assumption women make is that because a man may not express his feelings or he has difficulty when he does (think Hugh Grant in *Four Weddings and a Funeral*), he may not feel as deeply as she does. This simply isn't true. Men do feel things deeply but often contain those feelings more than we do and simply believe they're putting themselves on the line, unnecessarily, to express them.

It's important to remember that a man does have feelings, but they may NOT be the same as yours. Just as if you and your best friend were both in love, she may feel different aspects of her relationships are more important than the things you feel strongly about. We're all individuals.

The roots of our differences lie with our distant ancestors again. In our nurturing role, back by the 'campfire', we simply had to be in tune with the needs of our newborns. We had to know when their crying was over something basic, like tiredness, or something more important, such as illness. Likewise, ancient men had to learn to suppress feelings, particularly fear, when out hunting and fishing. They needed to concentrate on the task and couldn't be distracted. Feelings came second to the job at hand – quite the opposite of ancient women, for whom feelings were important. Understanding this can go a long way to accepting our differences. A big sign of his feelings comes from his behaviour – does he treat you well? Then he's got the right feelings!

Working With The Way Men Feel

Your relationships will be much smoother if you get to grips with some basic rules about his emotions. Try these:

➢ Men recognise they have feelings for someone new but don't always want to delve too deeply into these. Life is much easier if they don't feel pressured to talk about these new 'sensations'.

➢ Often men know they feel something but can't identify it – is it simply sexual excitement or do they really care? They find it harder to label their feelings. We can tell quite quickly if it's *lust*, *like*, or *love*.

➢ Strong feelings can provoke anxiety in men. Sometimes they choose to ignore them – and they may lose out in a relationship. Men may have more sexual partners in their lives but they fall in love less frequently than we do.

➢ Because they may want to 'ignore' strong feelings, they often don't have the relationship vocabulary to describe them. Keep it simple when talking about your new relationship.

➢ A lifetime of programming *not* to show their feelings won't be changed overnight. Even their mums told them, 'Big boys don't cry.' Why should they believe any differently? Coax it out of them.

➢ What you see is what you get. You may have a million wonderful emotions. He may feel only one.

➢ He may learn to open up with you – but don't drag it out of him in front of his friends!

➢ Ask what he's thinking and you may get an idea what he's feeling.

➢ Tell him your feelings in moderate doses.

One-Night Stands

If you're looking for love and a relationship, then you should avoid one-night stands. Only a small percentage of relationships blossom from a one-night stand. Having no-strings sex is absolutely fine if that's all you want (play safe!). However, one-night stands can have a high emotional cost. I've had countless women tell me they thought there was a special connection and so they had sex straight away – only to be incredibly disappointed when he didn't ring.

Why do so many men do this? Unfortunately, we're living in the REAL world, not the PC (politically correct) IDEAL world where no one is judged. Many men still judge a woman unfairly if she has quick sex. They figure she must be doing it with every other guy. So they're thinking, 'I'm not so special am I?' Really, trust me, many men have a fairly low opinion of themselves in this regard.

At the same time they're confident enough to take sex that's on offer and simply enjoy it. They're far more capable of having no-emotions sex and enjoying the physical side of a one-night stand. There are men who feel that one-night stands cheapen *them* – however, they're rare. A survey found that 98 per cent of single men would take sex that was on offer without too many qualms.

So you've been warned. If you want more than sex then don't have sex with him until you know what he wants too. Over time, it'll become fairly obvious whether he sees you as just a casual date or is really interested.

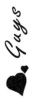

Men And Love

Funnily enough, we're bad at giving men a chance if they haven't leapt straight off our romantic checklist. Men are even worse at this! In some ways they're pickier about whom they fall in love with. Going back to their ancient roots sheds some light on this. Their genes tell them to spread their seed (that is, have lots of sex) but it's quite another thing to look after and provide for those offspring. So, somewhere in their genetic code they seem to be more wary of settling into a *love-thing*.

Knowing this means you have to be fairly subtle at sliding them into that *love-thing*. The better a man feels around you, the more likely he is to acknowledge deep feelings and fall in love. Of course, some men love a woman who's a challenge. However, most men want to enter a comfort zone that's probably reminiscent of how their mother nurtured them – but they'd never admit this!

So, the keys to engendering a good feeling around you are:

✓ Make things easy. Know what you'd like to do without being bossy.
✓ Be affectionate – but not in front of his friends, if that irritates him.
✓ Ensure you're not waiting for his call – but enjoy him when you're together.
✓ Laugh at his jokes! It's simple – men feel good when they think they entertain you.
✓ Show you care, but without seeming desperate.
✓ Once you've got this good-vibe going, he's more likely to start acknowledging strong feelings about you.

Men And Commitment

Even if a man falls in love it may still be an issue for him to *commit*. The '*C*' word holds all sorts of 'darker' meanings for him. Many men see it as a loss of freedom, sexual adventure and even youth. Being in love doesn't necessarily mean 'forever', but to commit – either to marriage or living together – well, this sends all sorts of alarm bells ringing. So, just as getting him to fall in love means providing him with a fun, inviting comfort zone, you need to be aware that getting him to the next hurdle also involves making sure it feels good for him.

Getting a man to the point of commitment is full of hurdles. One of their worst fears is that they might actually get so comfortable in this *love-thing* that'll they go from being, say, a *25-year-old guy-about-town* straight to a *middle-aged type*. That's scary!

The most interesting thing about men reaching their 'commitment threshold' (as I call it) is that it takes them longer to get there but – once there – they're less likely to dump the relationship than a woman. Women seek 70 per cent of divorces. Men, on the other hand, think, 'It's working OK, why go through the torment again of getting to know someone else?' Remember, commitment makes them vulnerable – so be gentle! Be confident – his thinking will catch up with yours, just give him time. Watch out for the signs that show he's ready – he'll open up to you verbally with time.

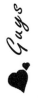

Guys

The Green-eyed Monster

Jealousy is a problem that most of us run into at some point. Recent research has shown that we have a 'jealous gene'. This probably served some sort of adaptive purpose in the relationships of ancient men and women. Feeling jealous was probably protective of the family unit and so sustained family groups against the odds when life was difficult.

We are not ancient women, though, and so need to rise above destructive jealousy. To start with, acknowledge any jealous feelings – they're OK. You're not superhuman. You may have them when some gorgeous girl gives your man the 'eye' or if he spends too much time with his friends. It's *how* you respond to them, and *what* you do with them, that counts. So, what should you do?

1   Identify what it is that actually makes you feel jealous in this situation. Is it that you're feeling 'ugly' – rather than the fact that he responded to another woman giving him a 'look'?
2   Once identified – sort it. In the example above, do something about the way you believe you look. If you two have gone out for drinks and you're wearing an old tracksuit and haven't washed your hair, you'll feel jealous of every passing woman with shiny locks.
3   Substitute a positive thought for your jealous thought. For example, 'I'm a fantastic person so what am I worried about?' Repetition works!
4   Tell your partner you're having an 'iffy' moment so that he knows you're trying to get over any jealousy issues. Hopefully, he'll be supportive.

Sexual Jealousy

Here are some *Golden Rules* on sexual jealousy:

❖ Past lovers are NEVER any good! Never start chatting about what your ex was like in bed unless you're saying how selfish and bad he was! If you beat around the bush and sound at all ambiguous, it's easy for your lover to misinterpret what you're saying and feel sexual jealousy. Anyway, why bring up an ex-lover?

❖ Beware of flirting when you're out together. When it comes to being 'territorial', men and women are just as bad as each other. For every story you've heard about a man getting possessive in public when he thinks his partner's being flirted with, there's another one of a woman getting jealous. We feel threatened when someone is interested in our mate. So it's best to learn how to deal with feelings of sexual jealousy.

❖ There'll always be good-looking men and women wherever you go. You both have to deal with this. Don't get involved when someone tries to chat you up. If either you or your lover gets a buzz from being chatted up, look deeper into this need. It's about reassurance for yourself. Be firm with yourself and don't get into tricky situations that upset your partner. Find things that boost your ego and don't involve flirting.

❖ And if your partner is jealous without reason – don't pander to it! If he rings ten times a day asking what you're 'up to' cut the conversation short or change it to something constructive. He's got to control this tendency, so set your boundaries.

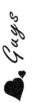
♥ Guys

Actions Speak Louder Than Words

A really clued-up woman knows that a man's behaviour speaks louder than words. We all love Hugh Grant in his mumbling, bumbling, *difficult-to-express-himself-type* film roles. But we tend to hate the real thing! If you're with a man who finds communication difficult, watch for the gestures that say he cares. They include:

✓ Giving you a pet nickname.
✓ Arranging a surprise meal or cooking for you.
✓ Giving you a surprise gift.
✓ Showing some sort of public affection – even if it's only a gentle touch to your back.
✓ Sending you jokey texts, e-mails – it shows he wants to make you smile.
✓ Ringing for no apparent reason – it means he wants to hear your voice.
✓ Opening up about problems at work.
✓ Introducing you as his girlfriend.
✓ Offering to help with something at your home.

Signs that he's not serious include:

❖ Giving his friends more attention than you.
❖ Saying, 'Let's take our time.'
❖ Saying he's not sure what he's looking for.
❖ You do most of the phone calling and 'chasing'.
❖ Never taking the initiative about what to do/where to go.
❖ Never talking to you about anything important – such as work, family.
❖ Making no effort to tidy his place when you come over – although he may simply be a slob!
❖ If you have a 'gut feeling' that his heart's not in it – listen to your intuition.

Retaining Mystery Is Different From Playing Games!

In these days of wearing our hearts on our sleeves, it's easy to forget that effusiveness about personal and intimate matters can be very threatening. Retaining mystery is different from playing games – those can put a man off. I like to think of it as revealing yourself slowly – like a sensual strip tease. What's sexier? Ripping your clothes off and lunging at someone while naked? Or slowly and seductively stripping away a layer at a time? It's the same with personal information – slowly does it – then he'll want to know even more! Here are some simple strategies to keep him interested until he's in love:

❖ Avoid the 'L' words – 'love' or 'like' – until he's really comfortable with you.
❖ Don't let him know you're having, for example, mood swings over work.
❖ Don't go OTT about past crises, such as telling him every detail about your parents' horrible divorce.
❖ If he's got plans, so have you! Even if those plans are to do a face pack.
❖ When he phones, give him five minutes. Don't let him think you've got all the time in the world.
❖ When people ring your mobile, don't tell him who's just called you.
❖ Space your dates at first. Twice a week for the first three weeks is plenty. Don't tell him what you're doing when you're not seeing him. He's not your keeper.
❖ Don't let him know that it took you an hour to get ready. Your personal habits are private!
❖ Don't discuss illness in detail unless it's something very obvious.

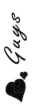

67

The Art Of Conversation With Men

Women have become so competitive that men now say they feel that they're in a competition when on a date! It's great that you're top dog at work, or a black belt in karate. But with a man you should be an equal – not a rival. Remember, men tend to have a 'need-to-know' style of communication – they may not want to tell you every little thing – so slowly, slowly! Try the following for cool, not competitive, conversation when first dating:

✓ Avoid the 'bulldog' phenomenon – if you disagree on a topic, let it go. Don't wrestle with it like a bone.

✓ Don't use your 'intuition' to always be right, saying, 'I know this because my intuition tells me.' That's the easy way out when you don't have facts to back your point.

✓ Avoid the 'broken record syndrome' where you repeat things. Research has found that women repeat themselves more often than men.

✓ Don't use 'verbal slaps' when you don't agree – such as telling a man he's 'silly' or 'doesn't understand'. Men take these things deeply.

✓ Great conversation is like a *gentle* game of tennis – not a hard-fought tournament.

✓ Never use 'shut-down' lines that stop conversation dead, such as, 'You wouldn't understand – you're a man!'

✓ Variety is the spice of good conversation, so cover lots of topics.

✓ Ask him what *he* knows about a topic. This is like giving him a 'stroke', generating love vibes.

✓ Watch your vocal tone. If you're warm, soft, and sensual you're more likely to be listened to – not shrill and demanding!

Have A Life

There's nothing sadder than a woman sitting by the phone waiting for a man to ring, or checking her mobile for messages every couple of minutes. Have you ever checked a line because you thought it might be malfunctioning? Most have, but this is really unhealthy for a relationship. Would you like to go out with a man who waited for you, like a doormat with no life?

I call this the 'Princess Syndrome' as, once upon a time (in the Middle Ages), princesses waited for their knights to charge by. Why do you think men would find the Princess Syndrome attractive? They don't. Word of warning here – a man who wants to control you will expect you to wait for his call. That's not healthy! Here are some tips to break the Princess habit:

➢ Force yourself not to answer the phone one evening per week. Be busy doing what you want. Period!
➢ Put a fun message on your answering machine. Not one that lists every possible place you might be found – that sounds like you're obsessive and overly keen to be found!
➢ Ask a friend to be your 'crisis buddy' – when you feel like ringing the new man in your life – ring her instead.
➢ Do not make silent calls withholding your number, at any time – ever!
➢ Do NOT drop plans you've made if he rings wanting to see you.
➢ Make the other things you have to do interesting – so you really want to do them and aren't grudgingly 'keeping busy' because you know you should.

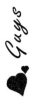

69

Dating And Your Friends

We have a terrible habit of dumping our girlfriends when we fall for someone new. This is something many women regret, especially when the guy's gone and her ex-best girlfriend doesn't really want to know. So you need to ensure you don't neglect your girlfriends when you fall in love. Try these:

> Make dates with her too – and stick to them.
> Keep any long-term plans you've made with her – like that long-awaited trip to Australia. The new man will just have to wait.
> Every time you text your new love, text her too.
> Try to get him to bring a friend along for a double date. Nothing serious, just four people getting together to have fun.
> If she already has a boyfriend, make up a double date with him.
> Never forget you can have both – a relationship and a best friend.

The other big problem – from the opposite direction – is *envy*. Sometimes you might find that your friends envy *you*, especially if they're not in love, or think you *always* get the guy, or maybe they liked him, too. How to prevent envy:

> Let her know how much you value her friendship.
> Talk to her about your worry that she's not happy with your new relationship. Hiding these thoughts makes them fester.
> Don't drone on about how wonderful Mr Possibility is – make sure your conversation revolves around things besides him.
> At the end of the day, if she has a big problem with envy – she'll have to change!

The Rule Of Three

There are three hurdles that the vast majority of couples face – I call them the *Rule of Three* – and they can make or break a new relationship. Let's go through them, so you know how they work:

Third Date If you make it past the first date then, by the third date, you'll probably have decided whether there is real interest *or not*. It's usually after the third date that women complain he didn't call. By the fourth date, they find they really start 'getting to know him' since they've made it that far. By the third date you can see past your initial chemistry a bit and not have your judgement clouded by it. So treat date No. 3 like the first – be on your best behaviour if you really like him. Don't let the side down.

Three Weeks Having made it to three weeks, this is when people start dropping their guard. You may suddenly find they have an irritating habit they've kept hidden. Or else something you thought was 'sexy' actually turns you off – such as his laugh! This is the point at which one or the other of you may back off, as little things take on a bigger meaning.

Three Months This is a critical time for 'big decisions' to pop up – and make waves in any relationship that isn't solid. You may want to hear that he 'loves you' because you feel that way. You may find that one of you is always spending nights at the other's home – so topics like 'moving in' come up. How well you discuss these things will determine whether you fall at this important hurdle.

Does My Bum Look Too Big?

There are some things we can't resist asking a man – even if we *know* we'll never get straight answers. Men find it really hard to walk that line between honesty and tact. They hate the idea of hurting a girlfriend over such questions but worry they'll be caught out lying. So give them a break! Think about it. The question, 'Does my bum look big in this?' is tantamount to him asking you, 'Does my penis look small?' How would you feel put on the spot with that question? It's really more about your esteem than your size! Men know we fret about our bums, so you'll really make him squirm. Here are some other questions that men find hard to answer and so you should *avoid* – or at least not ask them *directly:*

❖ Do you like my friends? You can ask this one only after a few months together.
❖ Do you like my mother? *Never* ask this one! Let this relationship develop slowly.
❖ Do you love me? *Never* ask this one – wait and see if he tells you at some point after the six-month mark. Before that and you're very lucky! Some men never can say those three little words – so do their actions say it for them?
❖ When did you *know* you loved me? Unless he's the rare soppy type, he won't be able to answer this. Men fall in love but can rarely identify when they knew. Unlike *us* – we can tell them the minute and second when *we* knew!
❖ Was your ex more attractive, sexier, funnier, more popular, than me? Don't even go there! He's with you now.

Your Intuition Radar

We were given a 'sixth sense', our intuition, for good reason – to sense danger back when we lived on the plain and in the jungle. *Real* dangers were around every corner and our ancestors paid attention to the feeling of hairs rising on the back of their necks. However, I find women today simply don't want to pay attention to their intuition.

What sorts of things does your 'intuition' tell you? Your intuition is like your subconscious policewoman. If you're about to ring the man you just met but you have this niggling 'suspicion' that you might sound desperate – listen to this suspicion. Your intuition has picked up all sorts of information about him at a subconscious level. Like a radar searching for 'signals', it has, for example, detected that this new guy is reserved. So ringing may frighten him off. We may choose to consciously ignore such signals but our intuition is a clever piece of our make-up trying to alert us to situations. Here are some more things our intuition radar tells us:

➢ The outfit we've chosen might just be a little over the top, so dress it down a notch.
➢ We're 'gushing' too much information about ourselves in our conversation. Tone it down and ask about him.
➢ We don't think he really fancies us. Your radar's probably noticed him eye-up every bit of totty that's walked into the bar.
➢ Finally, our bum *does* look big in this new outfit we made a rushed decision about – believe it, it may do.
➢ He's unreliable. Many women choose to ignore it when their intuition says this!

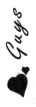

73

Your Dating Confidence

The more confident you are, the more successful your relationships! Research shows similar levels of confidence attract each other. If you lack confidence you'll subconsciously choose a man who also lacks confidence. His lack of confidence may come out in toxic ways, like: *1* Bullying you. *2* Two-timing you to build his own self-worth. *3* He may lie, cheat and undermine you – because he knows your confidence is too low to stand up for yourself. *4* He may simply be like you – and the two of you together forge a relationship where you both fret and worry about things, or get into a rut, and don't have the confidence to try new ways of relating or improving things. Here are the 'dirty dozen' signs that tell a man that a woman feels unworthy:

1   Shy and awkward body language.
2   Not saying what she wants to do on a date.
3   Picking at food – fear of eating in public.
4   Appearing eager to please.
5   Feigning interest in something – when clearly she's not.
6   Wanting to know every detail of his relationship history – she doesn't have confidence in the fledgling relationship.
7   Asking to be compared to an ex.
8   Gushing about her romantic successes – she's got something to prove.
9   Bragging about how many men are after her *now*.
10 Claiming she's not looking for anything right now. ('The lady doth protest too much'!)
11 Being overly flirtatious to prove she's a sex kitten.
12 Asking overly personal information about him. She's lost control of her tongue!

Building Your Dating Confidence Will Improve Your Relationships

It's vitally important to build your general dating confidence so that you meet the most worthy men and have positive relationships. You can choose to continue to run yourself down, expect little from men, and generally continue along a negative path. Or you can choose to raise that dating confidence. (Raising your *general* confidence is covered in Part Three: 'Chocolate – Life', from page 94.) Try these:

➢ To practise saying what *you'd* like to do with him, try saying what you'd like to do with friends and colleagues.

➢ Many women judge their 'date-ability' by their size. If they're large they think they have nothing to offer. You can choose to focus on your size or you can choose three attributes you have to focus on. (More on weight on page 120.)

➢ Stop trying to please men. Men love strong women so say things you mean, express your opinions and views.

➢ Don't allow bad past experiences to cloud your dating *now*. Select one good date from the past and remind yourself of this one.

➢ Seize dating opportunities. If the nice man in the lift at work suggests coffee – say 'Yes'. Even if you don't fancy him, it's good dating practice.

➢ Set goals, if, for example, you fancy someone at your gym. *Goal 1* – go and exercise next to him. *Goal 2* – smile at him. *Goal 3* – ask how to use a piece of equipment, and so on.

➢ Practise flirting by flirting with your local shopkeeper or the salesmen in a department store. Smile nicely, throw your head back, laugh and enjoy your interaction with them!

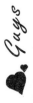

Getting Off On The Right Foot For A Relationship

Let's say things are feeling good. You've passed the second 'rule of three' – being together for more than three weeks. Here are some golden rules for building a relationship out of dating:

✓ Expect to have good fun and it might become a romance. Expect a romance and it's less likely to happen.

✓ Keep things in balance. If it feels like love it might be – but ensure you keep the rest of your life going so that you're not left high and dry after a month together. He dumps you – you're friends are angry, as you've ignored them, and you're behind at work, having spent four weeks daydreaming about him and his babies.

✓ Possessiveness is an ugly trait. The more you cultivate 'caring independence', the happier you'll be in each other's company.

✓ A great saying to remember when you're dating is: 'You attract bees with honey – not vinegar!'

✓ Both self-respect and respect for him are critical to developing a satisfying relationship. He's a unique human being – as you are. Respect his feelings, wishes and points of view – as you expect him to respect yours.

✓ A big mistake is trying to *change* him. If he's got faults you *hate* – he's probably not right in the long run. If they're little niggles, with time he can change those. You can change *yours* (yes, you'll have irritating habits too!) and accept the rest.

✓ Personal responsibility is critical to your developing love. You're responsible for your behaviour. He doesn't *make* you behave a certain way. You have choices, so make wise ones!

Married Men Myths

I'd be rich if I'd had £1 for every time I've been told a woman knows her married (or otherwise taken) partner is going to be all hers one day – and then it doesn't happen! Check out the figures: about 42 per cent of attached men admit to being unfaithful at some point. Only about 1 per cent of these ever leaves his partner. Not good odds!

Why women get involved with married men Usually they have low self-esteem and feel they only deserve 'crumbs'. It can be more complex – they might thrive on risk, excitement and hot sex. They may genuinely not want a full relationship – if so, why not have a part-time one with a single guy? Real intimacy frightens them and so their married guy will never be a threat. But love with a married man is not a game.

Why you can't trust a married man They're usually after sex and excitement, period! They don't want another relationship – they have that! What they don't have is excitement. You provide that – if you're stupid enough.

What to do Tell him it's over and give yourself breathing space. Do not be conned into letting him come over to talk about it. Get a crisis buddy – a girlfriend you can ring at times when you feel weak. Tell your mum – she'll talk sense into you. Don't take his calls. Look around the single scene – get out and find someone who can have a relationship – or just 'fun', if that's all you want!

Guys ♠

Coping With Infidelity

In an ideal world infidelity wouldn't happen. But it does and it's all too common. It's a myth that relationships can't survive it. Some simply survive it better than others. Here are the things to consider and try if one of you is unfaithful:

➤ Do you both want to work it out? If the answer's 'No' there's little hope.

➤ Don't make rash decisions in the immediate aftermath of discovery.

➤ If you're both committed to working it out, take a long look at why the person had the affair. There are so many reasons, such as stupidity, anger, revenge, feeling neglected, not thinking, sex, power.

➤ This is a time for honesty – otherwise it won't work. You've had the pain. Now you need to face the truths.

➤ Facing the truth does not mean having to reveal every last detail of the affair. Let the person who has been cheated on choose how much detail they want. But remember, once you've asked for detail you can't go back. There may be hurtful things in the detail. Think before you ask.

➤ Expect a variety of emotions – just like a bereavement. You've lost trust – this is tough, and you'll range through anger, despair, bitterness and utter disbelief.

➤ Do not keep throwing up the affair in every little argument you have. This is very destructive and tells the partner who's been unfaithful that you'll never forget. This gives you less of a chance to work things out.

Meeting Each Other's Families

When you take on him you take on his family (and friends!) too. You'd be naïve to think otherwise. Unless he's an orphan, you'll have to share him sometimes – as he'll have to share you. Here are some tips for playing happy families:

➢ Treat his mother like a rival and she'll become one. It's a self-fulfilling prophecy. Instead, encourage him to have a good relationship with her.

➢ You love him and she raised him so show her respect.

➢ If he has an interfering mother – for example, one who wants to make his decisions for him – talk about it with him. Present a united but caring front to her and she'll have her wings clipped.

➢ Never ridicule his family – leave that to him, if he wants to.

➢ That said, families can be strange. You don't have to spend time with his family if they're difficult or abusive. Let him know why you're making other plans when he goes there for the weekend.

➢ Agree how much time you'll spend with both your families and divide this in two so that each gets equal time.

➢ Alternate spending special occasions at each other's homes.

➢ Try to stay out of family rows. They happen but you should ignore them.

➢ Give him a list of his family birthdays so he can send out cards for his side and you can for your side. Nothing's more irritating than becoming the 'diary secretary' for both families – unless you like those jobs!

➢ All these rules apply to his family – and yours.

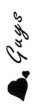

Guys

Keeping Romance Alive

Couples forget that the *only things* separating their relationship from simply being a strong friendship is romance and sex. Romance makes what you have that much more special. Like flirting, romance tells your lover that you want to *make him feel fantastic*. In a loving relationship romance is not forgotten. Try these:

✓ Create a love-tape of his favourite songs.
✓ Write a loving, affectionate, sexy note and leave it where he'll find it.
✓ Send him a text or e-mail spontaneously that says you're thinking of him.
✓ Ring him but only to ask about him – not to go through your shopping list.
✓ Offer to run an errand for him and come back with a gift.
✓ Guide him into a candle-lit bath where you massage his shoulders.
✓ Compliment him. Tell him, for example, that he looks great – *and make it genuine!*
✓ Ask him to help you set the table but then reach over, take his hand and give him a smoochy kiss.
✓ Make breakfast, lunch or dinner in bed for him.
✓ Surprise him at work with a lunchtime picnic.
✓ Ensure your next dinner is candle-lit with soft music – even if it's pre-packaged food.
✓ Don't neglect him; tell him you love him spontaneously. The list is endless . . . And he should be doing these, too!

Don't forget Some things should be kept private. Cutting your toenails, plucking your nose hairs, going to the toilet (unless you're both liberated about these things!), flossing your teeth, and so on, should be done when your lover's not around. It's hard for him to see you in a romantic light if you're crouched over the toilet seat hacking away at tough toenails!

Other Dating/Relationship Blind Spots

When it comes to dating and relationships, women have many potential blind spots. Here are a few I come across frequently.

What a man says and what he means Men view the goal as more important than the game so they often say things in a way that makes the point without all the detail and honesty. For example, 'You're too good for me,' means, 'I'm too good for you.' 'It's too soon after my ex,' means, 'I still love my ex.' 'I'm not looking for a relationship,' means, 'At least – not with *you*.'

Stereotyping We humans are quick to stereotype. We meet so many people it's easy (lazy!) to slot them into boxes. So we meet a man who seems 'shy' and don't give him another chance. What we don't know is that, with a little encouragement, he can be the life and soul of the party. Or we judge a man by his taste in clothes. Many men could benefit from the help of a good woman when it comes to dressing. So, within a few months he could look fantastic if he just had you to bring his style up to date. That's one thing you're allowed to change!

Missed chances Again, I'd be rich if I had £1 for every time a woman told me she missed a chance to go out with someone either because she felt nervous when he asked her out or she was having a 'bad hair day' and didn't believe he meant it. Go for those chances when they come along.

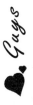
Guys

Tantric Techniques – So Much More Than Just Sex!

I've included this here, rather than in the 'sex' section, as Tantric practitioners are right to say that Tantric practices are so much more than just sex. Tantra says it's *the journey* you take together that's important, rather than the end. So with sex, orgasm is not the goal, it's enjoying the touching and being together beforehand that counts. Tantric principles are about connecting at all levels together. Here are some Tantric practices to try:

➤ Tantric breathing. To get in tune with your partner, sit facing each other cross-legged. Both of you place your left hand on your own heart and place your right hands on the other's heart. Close your eyes and relax. Eventually, you'll be breathing in synchrony. At that point, open your eyes and enjoy the intimacy of gazing at each other.

➤ Free your mind of fantasy and simply *feel* the moment together. As you touch each other, let your fingertips, lips, and bodies, simply revel in the moment. You should not be focused on orgasm.

➤ Whole body orgasm. Open your mind to approaching sexual release with a new attitude. *1* As your excitement rises, let your breathing *relax* – this is the opposite of what we normally do by breathing more quickly. *2* Clear your mind so that it becomes a blank slate. *3* Allow your muscles to relax – again the opposite of what we normally do when excited. *4* Keep moving together slowly and sensually. Gaze at each other and drift into orgasm, allowing all your sexual energy to flow through your relaxed body and breathing.

Babies And Relationships

Many women are shocked to find that their once rampant partner seems to go 'off' them after having children. He still lusts after women on TV but doesn't seem to want sex *with her*. This doesn't mean he treats her badly. But what he may have is the 'mother-lover' complex. I'll outline this phenomenon as I've heard so many women describe it.

What happens to some men after the baby's arrived is they can only see her in the role of 'mother'. Somehow he feels it 'tarnishes' the mother of his children to see her as sexy. Usually this happens with men from traditional families who tend to look at sex as something naughty. It can be very painful for a woman to suddenly be seen in one-dimensional terms. Try separating the two roles – parent and lover. Agree to no 'baby-talk' when it's your 'adult time'. Whatever you do, don't mention the children. Make a point of acting like you did in the years BC – before children. Start with romance and affection to rekindle things. This can be worked out!

Of course, the reverse is also true and sometimes women feel so overwhelmed by their role as mother that they've nothing left over to give to him as a lover. A woman may not like being touched when she's had a baby at her breast or clinging to her all day. Again a slowly, slowly approach helps. A couple finds that once they're getting more sleep, and adjusting to being parents, things will improve. However, if the problem persists, you should get checked for possible post-natal depression.

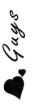

83

How To Argue Constructively

There are arguments in all relationships. Some people argue in a way that doesn't permanently damage their relationship. Try these methods:

➢ Sit down when calm and identify 'hot spots' that make you both angry. Most arguing forms a pattern around a couple of core issues. Plan how to sort out your differences.

➢ Write out both sides' points of view. See if there's middle ground you can reach and, if so, try planning for these. For example, if finances cause arguments see how your money can be managed so that you're both happier.

➢ Agree that on some topics you may not reach an ideal compromise but that this may be the best you can do – *so stop arguing!*

➢ If an argument starts despite following these points, count to ten before yelling anything. Counting to ten works! It gives your brain a chance to get in gear rather than be dominated by passionate emotions.

➢ If you feel yourself losing control, leave the room, saying, 'I'll be back when I'm calmer.' It's better to remove yourself when getting out of control than trying to stick it out. But don't use 'leaving' as a non-verbal threat to your partner – that you won't be back until you're good and ready – that's unfair.

➢ Never make sweeping generalisations such as, 'You *never* help me!' It's very rare that someone 'never' does something or 'always' does something. Avoid such statements as they put the other on the defensive.

➢ Rather than shout, 'You f**king b**stard!' try something silly like, 'You horrid booby!' so dispelling some anger.

Domestic Violence

The number of women who experience some sort of domestic violence is staggering. Some estimates put it at one in eight. Most women think, 'That'd never happen to me,' but it's surprising how domestic violence cuts across class and education barriers.

Often the woman is unaware that the relationship is heading that way as it can creep up in an insidious fashion. The man slowly isolates a woman from her friends and family. In this way he gains control over her ability to do things for herself. She also begins to doubt herself. Or it can happen abruptly: the relationship has seemed 'just fine' and then he suddenly attacks her. Often such a surprise attack leaves a woman reeling with fear, and feeling ashamed – so much so that she keeps it to herself. He may be very apologetic and blame it on a particularly stressful period. Any way it begins, domestic violence severely damages a woman's self-esteem. She may begin to believe that she deserves this behaviour. It also puts her health – and life – at risk.

Let me make this absolutely clear – no relationship should be based on fear. And an emotional bully can have just as devastating an effect as a physical one. No woman should feel threatened or menaced by her partner. And she should NEVER tolerate violence. If you find yourself in this situation and fear you can't talk to friends or family, ring the Refuge Help Line (0808-808-9999) or contact your local police station's domestic violence unit. If events overtake you, simply take your children (if you have any) and *leave* a violent situation. There are refuges around the country and the police will ensure you get to the nearest one that has room. Please do not feel that it's 'too late for you' and that you can't leave – you can.

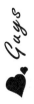

Guys

Knowing When To Let Go Of A Relationship

Sometimes we stick in a relationship that is well past its sell-by date. Usually we do this because we refuse to believe the 'proof' that we're unhappy. Instead, we cling to the myth that a little more love will change it. Optimism is great – but, at some point, if the relationship is bad for us, we have to face reality. Consider these:

❖ Do you feel undermined by your partner? Does he put you down in public and/or in private? Does he generally disrespect you? Some men act as if they really don't like women – and look for women willing to put up with their misogynistic behaviour.

❖ Does your partner have an alcohol, drug or other addiction that he is in denial over? Does he refuse to believe he needs treatment? Some addicts are no-hopers who'll never accept their problem. Others need a sharp shock – like a break-up – before they see sense. Once they've sought help, the relationship may pick itself back up and might work. If you have children with an addict you may be willing to take him back if he's getting proper help. But only if he's changing.

❖ Do you repeatedly argue over the same things, but never solve anything. Have you tried everything – yet your relationship never changes? Some people are gluttons for punishment and never leave unhappy relationships. You do have a choice.

❖ Does your partner repeatedly cheat on you? Do you keep taking him back? If you want this for the rest of your life – stay with him! If not, trade him in.

How To Tell A Liar

Humans tell little white lies all the time – these simply smooth the path of social interaction. For example, you may be late for something and blame it on public transport rather than admit you were dying for five extra minutes in bed. However, some people become chronic liars and manipulators of the truth – they make very bad lovers – and friends! What to watch out for:

❖ Practised liars may sit very still (*not* squirming in the chair) but look for tell-tale foot-shaking or finger-tapping as your conversation progresses.

❖ Liars often latch straight on to your gaze, rather than looking away shiftily.

❖ Watch out for pupil dilation and lots of blinking.

❖ As they speak, their voice may literally 'catch', almost like a small choking sound – they're literally choking on their lying words!

❖ Watch for defensive body language, such as crossing their arms behind their back, or across their chest, and leaning back – they're trying to back away from the conversation.

❖ Liars embellish with lots of detail – too much detail that they really don't need to give. Often it sounds impersonal – like it didn't happen.

❖ Listen to see if the pitch of their voice rises as they tell their story.

❖ A lying lover may over-do the innocent puppy dog look.

❖ They may pause at the start of an answer (as they think of an excuse) and at other points as they continue making up the 'facts'.

❖ They may get angry with your questions as their tension mounts.

❖ Watch for their eyes flicking away with each answer – a sign of discomfort.

❖ They may answer your question with a question to deflect attention.

The 'F' Factors – Predicting Whether It'll Work

I devised the five F factors to help predict whether your love will survive. They're based on the five areas people talk to me most about in finding harmony/compatibility or disharmony/incompatibility. Think about how these may affect your relationship:

Family background Research shows that background plays a large part in determining relationship success. If you have similar upbringings you're more likely to have similar outlooks. Opposites can attract but look closely and you may be surprised at the similarities. I'm an optimist and believe love can overcome wide differences in upbringing.

Friendship circle If you get on with each other's friends your relationship will be easier. But it's possible to tolerate each other's friends for the sake of your relationship, even if they're not *your* choice of best friends. This goes back to respecting the other's choices (within reason!). It's healthy to strike a balance between spending time together with friends you both enjoy, and separately with friends you both like individually.

Fanciability or – let's be honest – the 'Fuck factor'! Fancying each other at the beginning is easy! Where problems begin is when, for whatever reason, you stop fancying each other. Keeping the romance going, and trying the variety of sex techniques outlined in Part One: 'Sex – Lust' will keep things lively.

Financial agreement Arguments about money feature in something like 30 per cent of divorces. It's vital that if you have different outlooks you must compromise and *plan*.

Fun and leisure It's fine to have separate hobbies, interests and sports. However, the couple that 'plays' together tends to stay together. Find at least one shared interest!

Breaking Up Is Hard To Do

If it all goes pear-shaped and you're left facing a break-up there are eight key points to remember:

1 You can remain friends but you *don't have to be*. Being 'friends' after a break-up is some people's idea of hell, while others see it as incredibly important. Work out what suits you.

2 Expect the unexpected. One day you may feel angry about your ex, the next incredibly sad. Go with the flow and act appropriately, for example, if sad, ring a friend and don't isolate yourself.

3 Do something you always wanted to do but couldn't because your ex didn't want to. By doing something new you'll realise that you don't need your ex by your side.

4 Don't become, what I call, a 'break-up bore' – talk about your ex all the time and you'll think about him all the time. So talk about other things!

5 Don't look for love for at least six months. Dating is fine but rebound relationships can be disastrous for your healing – adding a whole other set of problems into the equation.

6 Care for yourself. Be aware of what gets you down – like your 'old song'. Switch off the radio when it comes on. Remove reminders so that you can move on.

7 Try to put things in perspective. You will love again. You probably loved before this relationship so why won't it happen again? Just don't worry about it.

8 Don't get involved in risky forms of revenge. The best revenge is to get on with life! And I'm talking about 'life' issues and considerations next.

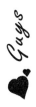

Guys

CHOCOLATE—

Life

You Always Have Choices

Why did I call this section 'Chocolate'? Because life *is* like a box of chocolates, to quote the movie character Forest Gump. You always have choices when opening chocolates! Making choices is not always straightforward. The choice you make doesn't necessarily lead to the outcome you want. For example, you make a choice, thinking it'll lead to one thing – the creamy caramel you want. But it leads to something else – a pineapple cream – yuck!

But is a pineapple cream going to kill you? No! Which is why I believe it's always important to make a choice and respond with an open mind to the outcome. Because what's the alternative? A life where you feel you don't have a choice? If you feel that way you're likely to get stuck very quickly when faced with the common problems of life – like making choices about work, family, relationships, and where to spend your holiday!

An important aspect of choice is realising there are often many choices you haven't thought of. The biggest tip I can give you to ensure flexibility when facing choices is to ask you to do one task. Think of the last choice you made, write it here:

I chose to _____ .

With hindsight list three other possibilities you could've chosen:

1 _____ .
2 _____ .
3 _____ .

With hindsight, people often say, 'Ah Ha! I could've chosen X, Y, or Z!' Turn that hindsight *into foresight* the next time you're faced with choice.

Chocolate

93

Why Does Everyone Else Seem So Confident?

It goes without saying that confidence is incredibly important. Think of confidence as being like the foundations of a house. The stronger the foundations, the higher it can rise, the more it can withstand weathering over time – and the more esteem you hold it in. Confidence and self-esteem go hand in hand. You need to strengthen your foundations! You're probably no more or less confident than the next woman. But if you lack confidence to live life fully you need to strengthen it. The first step is to identify why you lack confidence. Answer this, 'Have you always lacked confidence or is this something *new* in your life?' If you've always lacked confidence, explore family history factors to discover where this comes from. You can't change these but you can gain insight to help you move on. The main culprits are:

Overcontrolling parents When parents try to control their child's life too closely, the subconscious message that the child receives is, 'We don't trust you to get on with things.' This doesn't inspire confidence in a child.

Overprotective parents Parents who worry, with each cold or cough, that their child is desperately ill, or gasp each time their toddler trips and scrapes a knee, give this message, 'The world is a big hurtful, scary place – so be careful!' This leads a child to feel overwhelmed by the world.

Parents' own lack of confidence Research shows 'confidence' is the sort of personality trait that can be handed down in families. If your parent(s) lacked confidence, this becomes your role model for how you should relate to the world.

Losing Confidence Through Life Events

If your lack of confidence is relatively new, examine events of the last couple years to see if you can find something that shook your foundations. Even if you didn't see the event as such at the time, it could be the culprit that is undermining you. Here are some examples that shake people's confidence: *1* A bereavement you actually haven't come to terms with. *2* A break-up that dragged you down and from which you never fully recovered. *3* The loss of a job, even if you've found another since. *4* Less 'connectedness' to your friendships, through long work hours. *5* Severe illness; and so on. Answer the following, 'In the last two years my life's been changed by . . .'

_____

_____

Recognising life-changing events is an important step. Otherwise diminished confidence from a life event can erode your ability to face the next hurdle in life. A little self-doubt is a good thing – on occasion, it helps us take a healthy step back from making snap decisions. But when it stops us feeling able to conduct our lives the way we want to – action needs to be taken. High levels of self-doubt affects each choice we make, down to little things such as trying on ten outfits and feeling we look bad in all of them. Confidence is about trusting your judgement. When's the last time you trusted your judgement; what happened?

_____

Was the outcome positive or negative? If positive, reflect on this the next time you doubt yourself. If negative, reflect on one thing you can learn from it. For example, 'I can't always be right – but then *no one* is!'

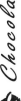

Chocolate

Confidence
And Self-esteem-boosting Goals

One of the first principles of confidence boosting is to set some goals for yourself to prove you can do things you've been shying away from. Accepting what you've done *well* bolsters your self-esteem. First, I want you to ask yourself if there's something you've been *thinking* about doing but have been putting off because, for example, you're 'not quite up to it'. Perhaps you've wanted to take an evening class or go for job skills training? Or even throw a dinner party? Let's tackle 'taking a night class' as an example. What do you need to do to achieve this goal? Make a 'need to do list':

1 Narrow the list of which evening classes interest you.
2 From the phone directory, make a list of colleges/centres offering classes.
3 Ring the most convenient one first and work 'outwards', making notes of when the classes are offered, their cost, how many people attend, how to register.
4 From all the information, decide which is the *best* option for you.
5 Book the class!
6 You'll hold yourself in higher 'esteem' once accomplished!

In looking at points *1* to *6* you can decide at what pace you complete them. If you're really lacking confidence you may do *1* and *2* one week and the others the next week. Small, manageable steps build confidence. Deciding you have to do *1* to *6* in one afternoon may overwhelm you if your confidence is on the floor. You decide at what pace to accomplish these and mark them in your diary. Good luck!

Prioritising Your Life

Another important element of general confidence is learning to prioritise what is good for your life. We frequently get bogged down trying to do too many things, with/for too many people. I'm sure you've known human 'whirlwinds' – never stopping for breath. Often this hyperactivity is a sign of low confidence because they *can't* prioritise. They don't have the courage to say to themselves, *this* comes first and *that* can wait. Such behaviour can lead to an 'all *and* nothing' approach to life – you give your 'all' to everything – get exhausted – and then give nothing! And suffer low esteem. When somewhere in between is just fine!

To prioritise, be brutally honest about your life. Make two, clearly defined lists. One ('*want to keep*' list) of the things you do that give some sort of pleasure, reward or return. The other ('*should let go*' list) of things you do that drain/stress you or make you unhappy. *Both* need prioritising. With your 'want to keep' list, rank each item in order of how important it is to you. Perhaps 'seeing friends more' comes above 'earning more money'. Both give you reward but, in your heart of hearts, one gives you more – so put it first. On your 'should let go' list, some items may be 'necessary evils' – like sticking with a job you hate until you've got another. But for each one you need to prioritise in what order they're dealt with. If you hate your job you need to plan goals (as per the previous page) to get yourself trained and ready to change jobs. Make your lists now and watch your confidence grow!

Chocolate

General Confidence And Self-esteem Strategies

Once you've set some goals and started prioritising your life, you'll find there are so many different ways to boost your confidence. The reason for this is that both our lives and our confidence are 'fluid' – changing and interacting with each other. For example, you're promoted at work – *boosting* your confidence – then find there are many new job requirements, which temporarily *sap* your confidence. A few weeks later, your confidence *soars* again because you've mastered the new requirements. So your daily life and confidence levels continue to influence each other: now that you've mastered this new position at work, you start to think confidently about making a whole new five-year work plan, scaling career heights you hadn't dreamed of before. You hold yourself in higher esteem knowing you can meet new challenges. Here are a few confidence tips that'll lead to higher self-esteem:

Focus on the positive You can choose to find the negative in daily life – or you can look for the good things that happen each day.
Self-affirmation Select your three best qualities – remind yourself of these each day. We all love compliments so compliment yourself!
Smile! You can leave the house with a frown or a smile – it's your choice.
Try something completely new Stimulate your brain by tackling something novel.
Encourage others Helping others do their best makes you feel good too!
Do something out of character If you're always 20 minutes early for appointments/meetings through fear of being late – force yourself to arrive *on time – not before.*
Telephone the person who always makes you feel good about yourself And tell them this.

Facing Fears

Fear plays a big part in almost every human problem. You'll recognise some of these: fear of being rejected, of saying the wrong thing, of not doing a good enough job, of being late, of doing something wrong, of being hurt, of getting angry and doing something you regret, and of not meeting *your goals*. Look at any problem you're experiencing and fear is often at the root.

The reason for this is fear is a basic human emotion stemming from when we feared wild beasts/fire/famine/attack/and so on, as hunter-gatherers. Fear plays a part in life to alert us to genuine threats (like walking down a dark street, your adrenaline increases so you're on your toes and alert – ready to respond to any danger) but gets out of control easily. How best can such general fears underlying our problems be faced? Identify, challenge and immerse yourself!

Identify the root fear of any given situation you're in or relationship you're worried about. For example, rejection.

Challenge it – what's the worst possible outcome for any situation causing fear, such as telling your boss that your report is going to be three days late. Will you be fired? No! Well, at least *I hope* your job isn't hanging by a thread – if it is, prioritise the issues bringing you to this point. Acknowledging 'worst' outcomes can often relax the fear.

Immerse yourself in your feared situation, such as, talking to your boss. Force some small talk with him or her. Plan what you'll say and then just do it! Getting into the feared situation often confirms the reverse – that it wasn't so bad after all.

Chocolate

Modern Life And Fear

Many elements of modern life jeopardise your ability to keep calm and fear at bay. For example, we're bombarded with information – mobiles, landlines, texts and e-mails, faxes, the Internet, and so on. These raise adrenaline levels, leaving us in a constant state of 'alertness' that isn't there for life-protecting reasons. This also leaves us prone to feeling as if 'something's about to happen' – even if it isn't.

Some suggestions to calm adrenaline levels, and to help diminish modern 'fear':

✓ Once a day, you can get away from 'it' by switching off your mobile, not checking e-mails, and so on, for a designated time. Again what's the worst outcome from doing these? The world won't end, will it?

✓ Prioritise incoming 'information'. Some people feel obliged, for example, to answer each e-mail in turn, regardless of importance. They don't bother introducing a way of prioritising (that word again!) e-mails. Develop a system of *A*, *B*, and *C* e-mails. *A*s are urgent. *B*s can wait a day or two. *C*s can wait as long as it takes. If you feel anxious, use an automatic reply saying, 'Thanks for your e-mail, it will receive attention in due course.'

✓ Being short of time increases adrenaline levels and modern fear – ask yourself why each meeting, or whatever, that you schedule has to be in person. Use conference calls and 'cc-ing' (copying) on e-mails, and so on, to avoid unnecessary meetings.

✓ Keep background noise levels down and play a soothing background tape during the day.

✓ Keep caffeine and sugar intake low. Phobias, of spiders, lifts, cars, whatever, are a special kind of fear and are dealt with on page 118.

Seize The Moment

As your confidence grows, making choices and taking action becomes easier – except when things arise *unexpectedly*. That is, when a 'moment' suddenly presents itself and you react in a negative, or benign, rather than a confident way. Most of us have what I call 'reactive habits' – we react in a manner typical of our personalities. This makes us creatures of habit and, for many of us, these habits prevent us from seizing the little moments of life that come our way. Think about the way you've reacted to the last three 'moments' that were presented to you. Did you: *1* Jump at it? *2* Procrastinate and miss the moment? *3* Say 'No' immediately? As I said earlier, it's important to seize moments *as they arise!* It's too late a day, or even a few minutes later to think, 'Why didn't I . . . ?' I'd be rich if I had £1 for each time someone told me they'd hadn't seized a moment. To become a 'Yes, please!' person try these:

1 Make your own moments. Off the top of your head, think of someone to ring and ask him or her to come with you for a coffee, see a film, or have a drink.

2 Visualise the last time a moment arose and you said, 'No'. Think about how it only took a second to say, 'No' and how you kicked yourself for the next two days! It'd take a lot less energy to say, 'Yes'.

3 Envisage the next time someone presents you with a moment. You smile and say, 'Yes please!'

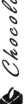

Chocolate

101

Killer Routines

Many women I speak to are scared of change. They want to keep their world an orderly place. You can be a slave to routine or you can learn to live life to the full. Of course, it's fine to have certain levels of routine in your life – particularly if you've got a young family. Routine makes children feel secure. (Although, to raise confident children who grow into adults able to fully realise their potential, they should learn while young that when routine changes – it doesn't mean panic!) Is the world going to stop if your weekly ironing gets done on a different night? Or you don't see your favourite soap opera? So how can you learn to believe that change is great? By learning to look for the positive ways to dump your routine and learn you can cope. Here are some ideas to get you started:

✓ Go to a different place in your lunch break today.
✓ Choose a different route home and look at the different trees, plants, architecture and people you see – savouring these new sights.
✓ Look out for new tasks at work to try.
✓ Buy something to cook that you've never tried before – an exotic vegetable or a different type of fish.
✓ Put your hair up one day if you normally wear it down, or vice versa.
✓ Go shopping and try on styles you normally wouldn't.
✓ Get a free make-up at a department store and ask them to go 'crazy'!
✓ Try one routine change each day.

Making Opportunities And Taking Opportunities

If you think failure to seize moments causes pangs of regret, then not taking opportunities causes real regret. Think of 'moments' as things that *enrich* your life and 'opportunities' as things that *change* your life. They're both potentially great. 'Opportunities' are simply on a bigger scale. We've all heard people say, 'The opportunity was there but I didn't have the foresight, courage, intelligence, and so on, to take it.' Key elements people use to increase opportunities are:

➢ Being aware of their surroundings – they tune in rather than tune out. So, for example, they spot a gap in a 'market' and think how to fill it. When I say 'market', I'm not just referring to business here – I mean any area of life. They can 'spot' when their boss needs to implement a new marketing system as easily as spotting the opportunity to meet the man they've noticed in the offices next door who looks absolutely gorgeous!

➢ By arming themselves with knowledge, they increase their chances of making and taking opportunities. Such people never stop learning about their life, which includes what's going on all around them.

➢ They're willing to share skills with someone else who can help them realise an opportunity – they're not selfish when they can see 'two heads are . . .'

➢ Finally, spotting that opportunity, that chance to change your life for the good, will become part of your life skills. You'll see things coming and have the courage to take them. Your homework: this month, spot an opportunity and decide how to use it!

Chocolate

Stress And Burn Out

Stress is a normal human response to facing life's hurdles – yet we've become a nation of over-stressed people. Unfortunately, we assume things like mod cons make life easier when, in fact, they complicate life. If you're getting texts from friends, e-mails from colleagues, and phone calls from your lover, as well as having to commute, compete with a shrinking job market, learn ever increasing technical skills, be the perfect partner, and so on, stress builds quickly. It's no longer a 'helpful' response but is becoming a habit.

Are you a 'stress addict'? If you get anxious/restless/irritable when every minute isn't about doing/achieving something, if you find it impossible to wind down even on holiday, if you have extremely high expectations of yourself always thinking you have to do better, and if you feel obliged to come in *under* deadline – even if it means working double hard – you may be 'addicted' to stress, or at least have what I call a 'stress habit'. Two million people now suffer from generalised anxiety disorder (GAD)! What else causes stress? Unresolved conflicts that bubble under the surface, lack of communication at work or in relationships, feeling you can't change things – helplessness, boredom (!), bereavement, divorce and other life events, and so on. To break a stress habit:

✓ Learn to delegate.
✓ Learn how to discipline your expectations of yourself.
✓ Seek help from others when needed (rather than feeling embarrassed to).
✓ Eliminate excess demands from your life.
✓ Ensure you have one full day off a week.
✓ Prioritise, as on page 97! If you can't break it – see a psychologist or counsellor – it's important! Unremitting stress leads to burn out – the new word for 'breakdown'.

Stress Busters

There are loads of stress busters but don't forget you should always look to *prevent* stress from building up by tackling the root of the problem. Here are lots of little tips to get you started:

➤ Use lavender oil. Sprinkle some on your pillow at bedtime, drop some in a steaming mug of water and inhale, or rub a little into your wrists.

➤ Do something with your hands – and it doesn't just have to be playing with worry beads! Model some clay, finger paint, knead some bread dough – even if you don't plan to bake it. Children always relax when doing such activities!

➤ Practise relaxation every day for at least ten minutes. Switch everything off, close your eyes and visualise a sandy beach.

➤ Watch your favourite comedy video and laugh – or simply recall a funny scene. Laughter is an amazing stress buster.

➤ Ensure your workstation is designed for the amount of typing/ paperwork you do.

➤ If you are a 'creative worrier' who always thinks of things you want to remember, keep a pad and pen near your bedside, in the kitchen, etc. I even have one in my bathroom!

➤ Get a self-massager or massage cushion if you don't have a partner you can take turns massaging with.

➤ Watch your caffeine and sugar intake!

➤ Get outside in your lunch break – a change of scenery helps.

➤ Have fun looking through holiday brochures. Even if you can't have a break this year – you can plan ahead.

➤ Get a good night's sleep (*see page 133*).

➤ Take up something completely amusing – art class, piano, clown skills, stripping!

➤ Avoid snacks of crisps and cakes; try a banana or fruity oatmeal bar.

➤ Try 'cherry plum' or 'impatiens' flower extracts, and valerian root, comfrey root, camomile, or cramp bark – in capsules or teas.

Chocolate

The Job Skills You Have –
Which You Weren't Even Aware Of!

Yes, boredom can cause stress. Boredom at work is a real problem. You spend more of life at work than elsewhere. Have you (or your boss!) squeezed yourself into a little box in terms of your potential? For example, do you call yourself a 'people person' or 'computer boffin' and then only do this? As we only use 10 per cent of our brainpower, people who excel at work, finding real job satisfaction, value flexibility in their job skills. Get out of your job skills box! Try these:

✓ I always recommend getting colleagues to do 'job swaps' for a day. If you've got flexible and forward-thinking managers, try to get them behind such a scheme. You may find you love doing someone else's job and can then look to train for such a move. But also such swaps promote good colleague relations – if you find out more about each other's work you'll also know each other more!

✓ Live your fantasy! Allow your mind total freedom – if you could do *any* job what would it be? No matter how far-fetched it seems. Would you like to be an author? A pilot? A radio show host? Someone's got to do these jobs, so why not work towards developing such skills in your free time? I have encouraged two friends to write/publish books and helped a couple of budding radio careers by giving friends slots on my programmes – because I knew they'd be great – and they said, 'Yes'!

✓ Take advantage of in-house training schemes. Even if it doesn't seem ideal – check out what you might learn.

✓ Use local adult education services.

Tackling A Difficult Colleague

We've all been there – putting up with those who make our job harder because they're unpleasant, lazy, malicious, and so on. I've got news for you – there are lots of things you can do to get along with colleagues. Never put up with sexual harassment, bullying, cheating, or lies from a colleague. First off, know your company's personnel guidelines for behaviour and complaints. But, as a start, try the following if your colleague's negative behaviour affects *you*:

➢ Make notes of when, what, and where their behaviour affects you.
➢ If it's anything you can approach them about, do so. But, again, make notes of when, how and where you do this.
➢ First, highlight the positives about your working relationship before mentioning what you see as a problem. Ask what they think.
➢ If this fails, and their negative behaviour persists, make an appointment to see your manager (don't just collar him or her in the hallway) and take your notes with you to discuss.
➢ If you don't get any joy from management or personnel, ring the Equal Opportunities Commission (0845-601-5901) over sex discrimination and pay-related issues. Go to your local Citizen's Advice Centre, or ACAS (0845-747-4747) for advice.

Key aspects of promoting good work relations:
➢ Never blow your own horn, except to your boss – who should know if you've met targets, and so on.
➢ Be generous with your praise for others.
➢ Head off problems before they grow – tackle the first signs with positive suggestions.
➢ Avoid gossip as much as possible.
➢ Don't get involved in other people's work conflicts.

Chocolate

Beating A Bully

Sadly bullying is rife in our society. From the playground to the office, to your family and relationships, you're likely to come across a bully at some point. Simply setting your boundaries and asserting yourself works with some bullies. However, with others the bullying can escalate as you try to stand your ground. Typically, bullies are angry, unhappy people who don't know how to communicate effectively and instead use aggressive tactics to get their way or upset their victim. Bullying can take many forms ranging from sly and manipulative behaviour to verbal aggression (the typical office bully), or it can be physically aggressive (usually younger perpetrators).

No bullying should be tolerated! You should seek help if setting boundaries or ignoring it doesn't stop it. If you don't deal with it, it can severely affect your self-esteem and create a cycle where you become the perpetual victim. Try these initially:

1   Point out to the bully you don't like their tone of voice or the content of what they're saying.
2   Make a note of any incidents of bullying so you have a record for personnel.
3   If it persists inform the bully you are making a complaint to personnel – most companies have anti-bully policies.
4   Ask a third party to 'chair' a meeting between you and the bully.
5   Do NOT be on your own with the bully.
6   If you are a parent and fear that your child is being bullied, explore ways the school can help you.

Some useful numbers and websites are: ABC – Anti-bully campaign (020-7378-1446), www.beatbullying.co.uk, www.bullying.co.uk, www.thesite.org

Tackling A Difficult Boss

If you want more than office *survival* but actually want to enjoy work, you need a good working relationship with your boss. It's easy to forget that the 'all-powerful' boss is human too – with all the worries and insecurities that go with that. The following strategies will help:

✓ If bosses make you nervous – picture them sitting on the toilet! Bringing them down to a human level helps you gain confidence in your interactions.

✓ Ask a friend to role play your boss and practise chatting to him or her.

✓ Also practise talking to other 'authority' figures, in less daunting circumstances, such as your tax office, doctor, and so on. As you develop communication with authority figures generally – it'll be easier with your boss.

✓ Learn *when* to tackle bosses – if the Friday pay roll stresses them, don't plan a problem-solving meeting then. Plan it for when they're happiest – Tuesday afternoons before the weekly tennis they love?

✓ Always promote positive aspects of work before tackling any difficulties.

✓ Asking for a rise: you can *never* be too prepared for this. Have evidence of all the good works you've done, goals you've met, *on paper* with a copy for *both of you*. Have a clear idea of the amount you'd like. It's no good asking for 10 per cent when others have only got 2–3 per cent. If you can make a *good* case for getting 5 per cent – you may get it. And think of other perks you'd like in lieu of extra money.

✓ Look professional!

Chocolate

Do You Say 'Yes' When You Want To Say 'No'?

Learning to assert yourself is a *valuable* tool for work and *any aspect* of life. Whether you find it impossible to say 'No' to the neighbour who borrows and never returns, your mum-in-law who hijacks weekends, the best friend who rings you at *all* hours, or the alcoholic brother who always needs help – any such circumstances will cause less worry if you assert yourself. People who aren't assertive worry that if they set limits others 'won't like them'. In fact, people respect you *more* if you do.

➤ Know and stick to your limits. You may adore your 'needy' friend but if your bedtime's midnight, be straight about *no* phone calls after that time.

➤ Believe your judgement. You're right – the person who borrows and never returns shouldn't be lent to. This doesn't make you a bad person.

➤ Give yourself permission to say 'No'. This doesn't mean you leave behind being a 'Yes' person to moments/opportunities – but you can't do everything! If you've been organiser of the last four charity fundraisers at work – and don't have time this year – let someone else do it.

➤ Know your rights so that you can return faulty goods. Do not be fobbed off by ignorant sales staff. Ask for a manager or customer services if something you've bought is faulty.

➤ When making a complaint, practise what you're going to say, keep calm, repeat yourself as often as you need to get your message through.

➤ Asserting yourself is not being aggressive. You shouldn't need to raise your voice or threaten anyone.

Make Your Mind Work!

You'll get more out of work, and more importantly, *life* if your mind is clear and alert. Just as a messy house can bog you down as you survey mounting trash, dishes piled high, and unsavoury smells emanating from sinks, so too if your mind is full to the brim with extraneous information – it'll bog you down. Here are some tips to keep your brain in top shape:

✓ Improving your memory will keep your brain sharp. Do this by putting it to the test regularly. If someone gives you a phone number, write it down and then test yourself until memorised. Same for any information – write it down (if your memory fails you!) but use your brain and try to learn it.

✓ Do brain teasers or crosswords each day. Even for just ten minutes, it'll get those brain cells firing. Any newspaper has these – so no excuses!

✓ Getting organised stops you draining your brain unnecessarily. Create a home filing system that's logical to you – and stick with it – so you can find tax forms, house insurance papers, whatever . . .

✓ Keep a list of all-important numbers taped to or keyed into your phone. Taking the stress out of finding, say, the doctor's number or your boss's mobile, will help you keep focused.

✓ Read nightly! A book stimulates the brain. Discuss it with others.

✓ Eat loads of oily fish such as salmon and mackerel – they're brain food.

✓ Keep set places for car/house keys, shopping lists, and so on. Chasing after them drains your brain!

✓ Always add lists of numbers in your head – throw your calculator out.

Chocolate

Get Lucky!

Many people believe that life is controlled by fate and luck. Yes, there are certain things you can't control – they're controlled by fate. For example, the weather and the behaviour *of others* on a more personal level. But the rest of life and how 'lucky' you are is up to you. Call it making your own luck, or simply behaving in ways that enhance your life – there are some key principles to help you. Let's turn to some classic sayings to help you get lucky:

If at first you don't succeed – try, try again! 'Lucky' people keep trying as they know giving up gets you nowhere. I'll use a personal example to illustrate. In 1996 I wanted to write magazine features. I went through women's magazines, one at a time, writing letters to the editor with ideas geared to their target readers. After the first twelve turn-downs (!) I finally got a reply (the thirteenth – who said thirteen is unlucky?) asking me for a sample feature. I've been writing ever since.

You're mistress of your own destiny! 'Lucky' people know that if you leave your life in the hands of others you won't get what you want. But if you take control and live how you want to – you'll reap many rewards. You make your own 'luck' by making your own decisions and reacting in the best possible way to other's behaviour.

Every cloud has a silver lining! 'Lucky' people know that just because something 'bad' happens, or doesn't go their way, they may learn something, find a new path, or grow in maturity through facing this 'cloud'.

Energise Your Life

Many women complain of a lack of energy. This can be due to stress – you've already read about de-stressing your life. It can be lack of sleep (coming on page 133). But it can also be the way you run your life generally. Here are a number of important considerations for re-energising your life:

✓ Sex! After the initial effects of oxytocin, released during orgasm, that make you feel sleepy – you're then rein-vigorated! Research shows that having sex twice weekly keeps people looking and feeling younger. Use it or lose it!

✓ Exercise! Exercise *gives* energy. Only *too much* exercise is detrimental. Ensure you get moderate exercise consisting of three 30-minute aerobic sessions per week plus 20 minutes daily of something else, like a vigorous walk.

✓ Flexibility! I'm not big on yoga but medical research shows keeping supple keeps you youthful and energised. You don't have to find a yoga class. Buy any book on exercise that includes stretching techniques to keep you flexible.

✓ Diet! What you eat determines, to a large extent, how energetic you feel. Food is fuel! A diet of pre-packed foods, high in sugar and fats, won't fuel your busy life. Ensure that you eat fresh fruit and vegetables daily. Drink water or fruit juices instead of fizzy drinks. Avoid fried foods that leave you lethargic. Eat slow-burning carbohydrates (pasta, brown rice, wholemeal bread) for energy.

✓ Do something childish! Swing on swings, fly a kite, watch your favourite childhood movie (*The Sound of Music!*) – these help you find your inner child. And children have energy!

Chocolate

Karma

Have you ever done something you regretted? Maybe had a go at a friend or snapped at a colleague who really *didn't* deserve it. Or maybe they did deserve to have their socks pulled up but not in the way you did it. Let's be clear, I don't believe in some mystical form of karma but about how your actions towards others make them *and you feel*. People forget that when they treat people in a 'not good enough' way they may end up feeling guilty or tarnished. So by 'karma' I mean that your actions *will* reflect on you and may come back to haunt you. Here are some ways to a kinder, more reasonable you:

➤ What's actually wrong? Dip you snap your way through your day because you'd rowed with your boyfriend? Anger's fine, but direct it at the right person.

➤ Identify your hotspots! Certain things push your buttons – know what these are and if someone brings them up – keep calm. Think before you speak!

➤ Accept blame! If you've done something that should be apologised for – give that apology. It actually makes you look like a better person and feels good.

➤ Flattery is fantastic! Always be the first to give compliments but make sure they're genuine. People see through false flattery but love real compliments.

➤ Listen and learn! We're all so busy that half the time we ask a question we don't even listen to the answer. If you're going to ask – listen. And make time to listen to people anyway.

Recognising Dysfunctional Behaviour In Ourselves

Do you often have a sense of 'Oh no, here I go again!' when doing something or reacting to someone? Remember the four behaviour 'profiles' (*see page 53*) – the Prima Donna, People Pleaser, Passion Victim, and Perfectionist? These 'P' behaviours cause problems not just with men but in your life *generally*. Make these 'personality profile' changes:

Prima Donna Put yourself in others' shoes. You can do this in your mind or *tell* the person you're interacting with them by trying to see things from their perspective. Feed back to them what you think they mean.

People Pleaser Your need to be 'liked' means you have little personality. Being the perennial chameleon, always fitting in with others, makes you pretty bland. Stop doing 'bland'! Practise speaking your mind within your family, then extend this to friends, and finally at work. You have a right to opinions, ideas, and feelings.

Passion Victim Try a daily meditation to relax yourself generally. Count to ten before you open your mouth. (OK – five – if you can't make ten!) When next faced with a situation that usually sends you into volcanic, 'passion mode', stop and think 'cool, calm, and collected' – people will actually pay more attention!

Perfectionist Ruffle your hair, don't line up those cushions perfectly, and ignore things that don't go exactly to plan. Lighten up on those around you – don't criticise friends (you'll have more!), family or colleagues unless you've got good reason, and then preface it with something positive first.

Chocolate

Recognising Dysfunctional Behaviour In Others

Women are too 'good' at putting up with bad behaviour – not just from men but from other women, colleagues, friends and family even. We've become the proverbial 'doormat' in too many situations, hoping for a change, expecting better behaviour next time. It doesn't mean that all who take advantage of this part of your nature are 'bad' people. Most people can be set straight if you're honest with them! First you have to recognise the sort of behaviour that you don't have to put up with and needs setting straight. Look out for these behaviours in others and try the responses shown:

1   Someone who always blames others for anything bad that happens. **Your response** 'Actually you're to blame for that situation.'
2   They are never wrong. **Your response** 'There's another side to this you know!'
3   They can't say 'sorry' when it's blatantly obvious they should. **Your response** 'You should apologise.'
4   They say one thing but do another. **Your response** 'You haven't done what you said!'
5   They lean on you but are never there when you need them. **Your response** 'Next time I need support, can I count on you?'
6   Someone who's always negative about others – a toxic person! **Your response** 'Can't you say something nice for a change?'
7   They're bossy, telling you what to do. **Your response** 'Next time, will you ask me if I want your advice?'

You get the picture!

Knowing When To Let Go In Life

Much of the time you *can* change people's 'toxic' behaviour, as just discussed. But if you repeatedly find that a person does *not* treat you with basic respect and kindness – whether a lover, friend, family member or colleague – you may need to let go. We all have different tolerance levels for 'bad' behaviour, varying from person to person. You may accept a friend who's a 'prima donna' (they've other great qualities). But not put up with the same behaviour in a colleague. Frequently we hang on too long. We're often frightened of saying, 'I've done my best and it's not worked.' If you're coming to the point of no return, try these final suggestions:

➢ Make a note of some examples of their behaviour – 'toxic' people have short memories.
➢ Choose a moment when neither of you are short of time or upset over something else.
➢ Avoid offering alcohol – you may think it'll relax you both but it also loosens tongues to say regrettable things.
➢ Preface your conversation with, 'I think it's time to sort out some differences between us.' This doesn't totally put all the blame on them and, quite frankly, you must share the blame for giving them repeated chances!
➢ Run your examples past them again without repeating 'You did this, *you* did that.' Simply spell them out factually. Ask for their thoughts on these examples.
➢ Finally, tell the person that this is their last chance – and *mean it!* If you don't mean it and back down they'll always know you'll tolerate their bad behaviour.

If none of these work then let go of it!

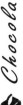

Chocolate

Phobias

Phobias are specific fears that are out of all proportion to the actual threat posed by the feared object/thing/situation. Arachnophobia (fear of spiders) in the UK, where you won't die from a spider bite, is *irrational*. But in the Amazon jungle it's acceptable as you *could* die from a spider bite! Common phobias include spiders, snakes, dogs, dentists, heights, public speaking, lifts, and the underground railway. Phobic reactions are common (about 16 per cent of people) although many won't own up to them (the guys!). How do you get one? Scientists have discovered a genetic connection but you can also acquire them from 'classical conditioning'. For example, you're sipping a fizzy drink, trip up, the drink fizzes everywhere and you develop a fear of canned drinks! Which explains why there are so many 'odd' phobias. Try these few steps to face your fear – I'll use arachnophobia to illustrate:

1. Define your fear carefully. What elements scare you – the look of the spider, the way they 'skitter', or their webs?
2. Rate from least to most scary 'spider' situations. Least scary – knowing a dead one's in the room. Most scary – one dropping on your pillow.
3. Start to 'desensitise' – building to more feared situations. First you look at a drawing of a spider. Next, visit a museum to see dead ones in displays. Third, you see live ones in protective cages at the zoo, and so on.
4. At the same time, practise deep breathing and visualising success!

Helpful organisations: Triumph Over Phobia (01904-610-202), National Phobics Society (0870-7700-456), No Panic Help Line (01952-590-545).

Adult Survivors Of Abuse

There are many adult survivors of abuse of different sorts – physical, emotional, sexual and neglect (that's abuse too). The One-In-Four Centre in London (020-8697-2112) states that as many as 25 per cent of adults have survived childhood abuse. This is staggering! Too frequently, sufferers exist in a silent hell, believing that they're to blame for the abuse. This is absolutely NOT true and 'survivors' *know* this at a *rational* level. But, at an *emotional* level, the guilt and shame arising from abuse are extremely difficult to rationalise.

The effects of childhood abuse are far reaching. Many 'survivors' find trust impossible as they've learned from childhood that if you can't even trust your parent (or other family member abuser) then whom can you trust? Many are self-destructive – continuing the pattern that seems familiar to them – that is, living with pain (emotional, physical and sexual). Many turn to excessive drinking or drugs in an attempt to block out the past. And, finally, some go on to be abusers themselves.

Some survivors grow into emotionally 'able' people through sheer force of character, and/or having the 'luck' to have relationships with people who are understanding and supportive. However, many need professional help to achieve happiness. If you're NOT coping with scars from past abuse, ask your GP for a referral to a psychologist/counsellor trained to work with adult survivors, or contact The British Psychological Society or the British Association for Counselling and Psychotherapy for recommendations. In the meantime, try this help line for support: Emerge Help Line (01543-576-174). Good luck! You WERE a victim as a child, now you ARE a survivor!

Chocolate

Mirror, Mirror — How Do I Look?

The diet industry is a £multi-million affair. If diets worked people would go on *one,* and *one only*, never needing another. But research shows that 20 per cent say they're always 'dieting', 39 per cent of women think about 'weight' daily, and 50 per cent of women have tried a diet. Only 25 per cent are reasonably happy with their weight. Genetic research shows 3–4 per cent of obese people have a 'fat gene' making them retain weight. If you're unhappy with your weight, you need to face the hard facts: for 96 per cent of you, how much you eat (intake) and how much energy you expend (output) determines your weight – not a gene! If you snack all day and don't leave your desk, your intake-output ratio is obviously poor! It's easier to say, 'I've got a slow metabolism so I can't shift weight!' than to say, 'I've got to eat less and do more!'

Face reality and do something about it or see *no change!* Check your Body Mass Index (BMI) – divide your weight in kilograms by your height in metres squared. The answer should be between 20 and 25. To a great extent, how you look is about how you *feel!* If you feel bad, sad, mad or lonely, you're more likely to comfort eat. Use all the esteem-boosting advice in this book plus:

1   Acknowledge your 'other self' not just your 'fat self', for example, 'I'm loving!'
2   Identify food 'triggers' that send you running for snacks, such as if your lover snaps at you or your boss criticises.
3   Make a list of these triggers.
4   Work out new strategies for reacting to these rather than eating. Tell your snappy lover to be more respectful. Ask your boss what you're doing right. Then phone a friend, take up a hobby with your hands, take a brisk walk, join a gym – but don't allow your trigger to send you to food!
5   Put portions on smaller plates – they look bigger.
6   Take B-complex, magnesium and chromium; some overeaters are deficient. Ring the Obesity Life Line (01477-544-344).

Eating Disorders

Sadly, some women get so hung up on their weight that it takes over their life. The most famous eating disorder sufferer was the late Princess Diana and I applaud the day she owned up to her eating disorders. It showed they can happen to anyone – even the most glamorous-looking women, who seem to have it all. And evidently about 10 per cent of women are borderline cases – all this dieting behaviour leads to a chronic situation in which they're at risk of damaging their health.

There are many reasons why some women are prone to eating disorders while others aren't. Again, genetics seems to play a part – but that doesn't explain the whole picture. Certain personality traits, such as 'perfectionism' coupled with wanting to 'please others' have been implicated. Also, a high rate of depression and anxiety are associated with eating disorders. And coupled with life stresses, when a woman's vulnerable, eating disorders strike. But it's not just women as now 10 per cent of those treated for eating disorders are men.

If you're 'starving' yourself, or secretly bingeing and purging (vomiting or taking laxatives), or an extremely 'faddy' eater, you should seek help immediately. Eating disorders have the highest mortality rate of any psychiatric disorder, with a reported 5 to 10 per cent of sufferers *dying*. This is a terrifying figure. Please do NOT be ashamed to seek help from family or friends, tell them – and then get yourself to your doctor. Try these help lines: The Eating Disorders Association (0845-634-1414) and Over-eaters Anonymous (07000-784-985 – for those who overeat and then vomit as a result).

Chocolate

Bad Hair Days And Human Intimacy

On a less serious note, many of us may not get depressed or fall prey to eating disorders but we all have *bad hair days* when we feel 'ugly' inside and out. Part of the ability to achieve true intimacy with friends, family and lovers, is to be able *to admit* when you're having a 'bad hair day'. Too many women worry they'll be rejected or ignored, particularly by romantic partners (rather than friends), if they own up to feeling bad about themselves. But, for whatever reason, we all have these days and that's when we need a hug! How to improve intimacy:

➢ Intimacy is a two-way street. The people you want to let in on how you're feeling need to be receptive. If they're in a bad mood or stressed out, too, they aren't the right ones to turn to at this moment.

➢ Attaining deeper intimacy consists of making step-by-step self-disclosures. Self-disclosure is like peeling an onion – slowly, layer by layer, you get to the core. Hopefully, the person you're relating to feels trust building between you and also starts to make step-by-step self-disclosures. But if you 'flood' someone, with whom you're trying to build a deeper connection, with *everything* that's in your heart and soul he or she may back off.

➢ When letting others in, tell them why you've chosen to talk to them – that you trust them and feel close already *or* want to feel even closer. Even partners should be reminded how much they mean to you at these moments.

➢ Don't let fear of rejection stop you reaching out when you're feeling bad!

➢ Be good to *yourself* on 'bad hair days' – relax, nap, see a movie.

Obsessions And Compulsions

Many women fall victim to obsessions and compulsions and often don't understand what's going on – or else keep them hidden through shame. Obsessions are thoughts, feelings, memories, beliefs that you can't get out of your mind – you *obsess* over them. For example, you may obsess over the way you write reports at work to the detriment of getting them in on time.

Compulsions are behaviours that you feel compelled to carry out – the choice feels like it's out of your control. Like checking you've turned the gas off ten times, or washing your hands five times before preparing meals. There's an obvious link between obsessions and compulsions. If you obsess about the gas exploding – you'll be compelled to keep checking it. So there are always obsessive thoughts underlying compulsive behaviours *but* people don't always act compulsively on obsessive thoughts. They may have the thoughts but not act on them.

Obsessive Compulsive Disorder (OCD) affects about 3 per cent of the population. OCD takes over someone's life completely and can prevent them from carrying out even the simplest responsibilities, such as leaving the house to shop, or holding down a job, or keeping a relationship. For others, their obsession/compulsion may be borderline. They may struggle with daily obsessions that are distracting, or compulsions that are time consuming, but still manage to get through their day. Excessive stress can tip this delicate balance and plunge the person into OCD. It's treatable by breaking the cycle step by step – so get help. Ring OCD Action (020-7226-4000) or Mind Information Line (020-8519-2122) for advice.

Chocolate

Sibling Rivalry And Family Rows

Families – they're there to love and support you, encourage you and nurture you, right? Wrong! Look at any family and you'll see rifts, fallings out and tensions. Except for the mother and father (who chose each other), families are a group of people thrown together by chance, all with individual personalities, but still expected to be 'best friends'. You do NOT choose your siblings as you would a friend. So it's a random event if you actually get along. You wouldn't expect to like everyone at a new job, would you? No! So why do we expect this of members of our family with their very different personalities? Accepting this one BIG fact improves your chances of getting along. Other things to accept:

Take turns Your parents want to give you all attention – even as grown ups – so accept sometimes one sibling or another will need/get more, for whatever reasons.

Step out of childhood roles Nothing's more frustrating than interacting as you did as children. You're now adults, so break the habits from childhood, such as, that the 'baby' *needs* advice – she may have her own family now. Or the 'eldest' *knows* everything – he may not know *anything*!

Don't compare Just because you're raised in the same family doesn't mean you're all going to have the same earning potential or lifestyle. Just as you wouldn't compare such things with friends – don't shove your siblings' noses in the fact that you earn more.

Envy And don't envy your siblings if they seem to be doing better!

Forgive and forget Move on from rows as quickly as possible.

Becoming A Parent

As mentioned on page 10, having a baby changes your relationship. Accidental conception aside, no one should enter parenthood without careful consideration. A child is for life and not just for Christmas! Here are some reasons NOT to have children:

➤ It'll solve your relationship problems. Babies are NOT bandages for you two.
➤ You think the baby will give YOU love. No, you should love yourself *and* your baby – a baby can't fill up any emotional 'black holes' you have.
➤ All your friends have them. Babies are NOT fashion accessories.
➤ You've got nothing in your life, so why not? A baby isn't a 'hobby'.

Parenthood is never easy but if you both know you're taking on a '29/8' commitment (and I don't mean 24/7 – a baby can make the week seem very long!), feel able to give up all your free time and work, too. If you're ready to be self-sacrificing – then go for it. Here are some baby 'Dos' and 'Don'ts':

➤ You *can't* give too much love but you *can* stop their independence by fretting over every move they make.
➤ You *can't* give too much attention but you *can* overindulge them with toys.
➤ *Accept* your baby for their own personality and *resist* comparing to others.
➤ Don't panic with each cry, just be there and learn what their little noises mean.
➤ Your hugs and kisses mean more than any flashy new toy.
➤ Set boundaries so they know how to respect others.
➤ Learn together how to be parents – take the best bits from your two ways of thinking about childcare!

For help and support: Parentline Plus (0808-800-2222), Meet-a-Mum (01525-217-064).

Chocolate

Making A Life Plan

After my divorce, I realised how thwarted I'd been as an individual so I resolved to set some life goals that I really wanted to accomplish. My personal life goals then were: *1* Be happy in a new relationship (I'm much happier in couple-dom than as a single – that's just me and I accept that!). *2* Be a black belt in karate. *3* Study psychology at a deeper level. *4* Write a book in the next five years (it took seven – so what?).

You may think, 'What a crazy collection of goals!' But life goals, dreams and aspirations are fantastic as long as you *plan* how to achieve them. These are bigger than the goals I talked about earlier. These give you an overall life plan. Life is short – start knowing what you want to do and where you want to be. Then have the flexibility of mind to accept what *actually* happens. Any of us can sit back and long to be Catherine Zeta Jones with children, awards and a doting (and rich!) husband. But if you keep *sitting* and dreaming – nothing will happen! I call it 'The Essential Life Areas Pyramid'.

1 Select the most important areas of your life – probably five or six of these, such as, work and personal relationships. Rank these in order of importance to you.

2 Look at each one and plan where you want to be with them in *five years'* time. Psychological research shows that five-year increments are key to whole-life changes. For example, it took me one year to plan *how to do* my post-grad studies and four years to *complete* them.

3 Allocate three to five hours per week working towards these, giving most of this 'pyramid' time to your top couple of essential life areas.

Bereavement

The only sure fact of life is that one day you, I, and everyone else will die. Your first experience of death may be that of a beloved pet or grandparent. There's so much fear of death that it prevents many from grieving in an emotionally healthy way.

Grieving is important because people who don't or can't grieve end up with all sorts of psychological anguish, which may lead to destructive behaviours, such as drinking too much to blot out their loss, or an inability to make close emotional bonds in future. And sometimes their life literally stops. There's no one right way to grieve. At the end of the grieving process it's important to feel you've 'internalised' your loved one – you feel them in your heart in a positive way. You can laugh to yourself and think, 'Mum would've loved this!' Typical feelings/grief reactions:

❖ Numbness during the early stages.
❖ Anger at the departed for 'leaving' you.
❖ Guilt over any unfinished business.
❖ Desperate pain and sadness knowing how much you've lost.
❖ A sense of being out of sync with time and others.
❖ Feeling like your life's on hold.

Certainly, in the immediate weeks after the death of a loved one, you may not function well at all. If, however, you don't notice things changing after the first month or two – for example, you don't feel anything but pain or anger – then get in touch with Cruse, the bereavement advice organisation, or a local support group. Honour your loved one's life in little ways and don't feel guilty when you're moving on – your loved one would want you to.

Cruse (0870-167-1677), Survivors of Bereavement by Suicide (01827-830-679), Child Death Help Line – for the loss of a child of any age (0800-282-986), Bereavement Register – for the removal of loved ones' information from data bases (www.the-bereavement-register.org.uk).

Chocolate

Alcohol

The figures are amazing – we now have two million alcohol-dependent people in this country! There are more than 33,000 alcohol-related deaths per year. In the 18–24 age group, women are drinking at dangerous levels, twice as much as men! Drink-related problems also cause the loss of fifteen million working days in industry. It's predicted that if drinking-related behaviour doesn't change, the NHS will 'collapse'.

Alcohol abuse takes many forms. There are those who binge on Friday/Saturday nights, those who drink more than three units per day, and those who go on occasional benders as a reaction to stress. Many women don't realise how vulnerable they are to damaging their bodies when keeping up with 'the men'. We don't process alcohol as efficiently and we weigh less. It's good policy to note how much you drink/how frequently and learn to have fun without getting plastered! Avoid drinking to relieve stress, to sleep better (a little too much alcohol has the reverse effect), to overcome nerves – these reasons lead to problems. Be aware of excess alcohol in your family, too. A unit is a small glass of wine of standard measure or half a pint of medium-strength beer (not one of the strong varieties). It's often hard to measure what's in your drink. Pre-mixed cocktails often contain one-and-a-half measures of spirits, and wine-glass sizes vary tremendously between establishments.

Government guidelines have changed but at this point you should not drink more than two to three units per day (with at least one alcohol-free day per week). It's a fallacy to think that saving up your units during the week to drink sixteen on a Friday night is safe – it's very damaging. There are many help and information lines to try, here are a few: Alcoholics Anonymous National Help Line (0845-769-7555), Alcohol Concern (020-7928-7377), Drink Line (0800-917-8282), Drug and Alcohol Help Line (01372-743-434).

Drugs And Other Addictions

People can get addicted to practically anything including work, sport, self-mutilation, and all sorts of drugs. It's harder to put correct figures on other addictions, such as drug abuse, as much is hidden. Suffice to say that drugs and other addictions also pose an enormous problem to society in terms of mental health, safety and lost days at work.

What makes an addiction? Well, there are various criteria that define when something has become an addiction, such as when the drug abuse/behaviour (such as sex addiction or self-mutilation) has started to jeopardise sufferers' emotional or physical health, their relationships, and/or their work. Addicts may begin to lie and use subterfuge in order to carry on their addictive behaviour. They may also be in denial and not believe 'they have a problem'. As the addiction grows they are more and more detached from the reality of their situation, losing friends, work, relationships, money, health and well-being along the way. Often addicts don't start recovery until they hit the proverbial 'rock bottom'. This is the turning point where one direction may mean death or total social exclusion, and the other direction is 'up'. Get yourself help! It takes courage to admit that you're an addict. Finding that courage and reaching out to friends, family and professionals will be a lifesaver. If you've no friends or family left, go straight to your doctor, ring the numbers below or look for a support group for your addiction. Many of the addiction clinics treat all addictions. Get the help you need now!

Narcotics Anonymous (020-7730-0009), Addaction (01582-732-200), Getting Off Tranquillisers (0151-932-0102), www.thesite.org

Chocolate

Smoking

Smoking is a terrible, deadly habit. Research shows that the vast majority start smoking before the age of 21, suggesting that it's the young who believe the myths – that it's sexy, cool, and grown up. If you haven't started by 21, there's very little chance you'll start. New research shows some young women smoke to 'stay slim', believing that cigarettes suppress your appetite – which they do to a certain extent. But once you're home, your appetite comes back with a vengeance, meaning you eat *larger* meals! Smoking is *not* sexy. Female smokers are less orgasmic and male smokers have up to four times more erectile dysfunction! To give up, try these:

1   List all 'negatives' about smoking – costs, illness, bad breath, and so on.
2   List the positives of stopping – what you can buy, longer life, and so on. If you've children, include 'setting a good example' and living long enough to see *their* children.
3   Set a 'stopping' date – NOT a 'give up' date. Saying you're 'giving up' makes it sound like you're *losing something positive* which you aren't. You're *stopping* something *negative*.
4   Before that date, get rid of ashtrays, lighters, smoking para-phernalia.
5   Enlist crisis buddies – tell them you're stopping and ring them for support.
6   Start new 'finger behaviours' – you'll miss the stuff that goes with smoking – so get worry beads, notepads and pens – anything to keep those fingers busy!
7   Suck ice, pick at fruit, chew gum (discreetly!), whatever it takes to keep your mouth busy but not take in too many calories, if you fear weight gain.

Seek advice from your doctor – there are smoking cessation programmes available for some smokers on the NHS, and you may be able to get nicotine-patch prescriptions from your doc. Ring the NHS Smoking Help Line (0800-169-0169).

Depression And You

Research estimates that almost 25 per cent of adults experience depression at some point in their life. 'Reactive' depressions – due to events such as bereavement, job loss or divorce – are common. However, chronic depression is less easily understood. Sometimes depression appears along with an event (such as divorce) but doesn't go away afterwards. At other times the problem can build up slowly until the person has full-blown depression. There are many possible symptoms, which can vary between individuals, including lethargy, excessive sleep, or sleeplessness, early waking, lack of appetite, food cravings particularly for sugars and carbohydrates, irritability, lack of emotion – feeling 'blank' or numb, feeling deep sadness and despondency, loss of interest in hobbies/work/sex.

Treatment includes counselling, medication, or a combination of the two. Left untreated, depression can be 'life threatening' as higher rates of suicide occur in depressed people. Counselling often involves cognitive-behavioural therapy (CBT). This looks at changing irrational thinking and introducing new, positive behaviours. *Seek help* and try these:

✓ Identify irrational thoughts, such as, 'I'm a failure as I lost my job.' Replace with positive ones like, 'I've had job success before and I'll get new skills training!'
✓ Take some exercise (even just a walk) to get the blood flowing.
✓ Eat at regular times, even if you don't feel like it. Include mood-boosters such as bananas, oily fish and carbohydrates.
✓ Avoid caffeine, excess sugar and alcohol (a depressant!).
✓ Visualise happy times and getting *these back*.
✓ Choose to see the positive side.
✓ Give yourself one treat daily – believe you deserve it!
✓ Talk to people without shame – you're not alone! Depression Anonymous (01702-433-838), Depression Alliance (020-7633-0557), Seasonal Affective Disorder (SAD) Association, if you suffer the winter 'blues' (01903-814-942).

Chocolate

Rape And Date Rape

Sexual violence of all types against women is sadly all too common. Home Office figures state that the police recorded 7,017 cases of rape in 1999, but estimates put the real figure at over 60,000 for that year. Due to the traumatic nature of rape many women choose not to report it. That is a personal choice; however, all women who've been the victim of sexual violence should seek the help and support they *deserve*, and be screened for STIs. Many victims experience a sense that rape was somehow 'their fault' even though clearly this is *not* the case; talking it through with a rape counsellor will help the victim understand this. It is rape whether perpetrated by a stranger or someone known to you. Rape can occur on a date, within a relationship or as a random or planned attack. Here are a few tips to protect yourself against rape:

1   Never accept a drink from a stranger, and *never* leave drinks unattended. 'Date rape' drugs like Rohypnol are colourless, tasteless and can render you unconscious.
2   Also beware of male-female teams who perpetrate rape – beware of accepting drinks from unknown men or women.
3   If someone makes you feel uncomfortable, trust in your intuition – a powerful tool!
4   Do *not* get incapacitated through alcohol or drugs.
5   Plan travel to ensure safety, and only use licensed taxi cabs.
6   Stick with friends and ensure you *all* get home safely.
7   Take a self-defence class.
8   Carry a rape alarm.

If you have been raped, call the Rape Crisis Federation Help Line (0115-934-8474), which can direct you to local support, or the National Victim Support Line (0845-303-0900), which will also help you find sources of local help, if these aren't in your local phone directory. Some groups offer support to any rape victim while others specialise in helping younger victims.

Nightie Night – Get A Great Night's Sleep

The benefits of a good night sleep are enormous. Poor sleep has been blamed for: *1* the inability to fight off illness, *2* keeping depression hanging around, *3* causing accidents at work, *4* lack of interest in sex, *5* low energy and general apathy. Most people require 7–8 hours nightly. But this varies, so get in tune with what you need! How to sleep your way to great health:

➢ Get a bedtime routine that's *restful* – a warm bath, relaxing book, camomile tea, and quiet lighting.
➢ Make sure your room is not so warm that you toss and turn, or so cool that it keeps you alert.
➢ If you're an anxious person, don't watch police/violent TV at night.
➢ Don't drink caffeinated drinks after 3 p.m.
➢ Eat a light evening meal.
➢ Don't exercise after 8 p.m. – high heart rates make it harder to sleep.
➢ Don't drink more than 2 units of alcohol per evening – more and your body goes into 'rebound' where your metabolism speeds up as the alcohol clears your system and you get an energy surge, waking you at 4 a.m.).
➢ Keep weekend sleep patterns similar to weekday routine. If you rise at 7 a.m. during the week and sleep until noon at weekends this is detrimental to your body clock.
➢ Drop some lavender oil on your pillow or place a mug of steaming water with lavender dropped in on your bedside table.
➢ If you worry you'll forget something during the night, keep a 'security' pad by the bed to jot down ideas as they come to you.
➢ Visualise a soothing beach scene with a warm sun shining down on you.

Chocolate

The Menopause

The most common definition of menopause is cessation of the menses (your periods and ovulation) for a year, usually occurring between the ages of 45 and 60. The whole process of menopausal changes can last from five to fifteen years. People once assumed the 'change' occurred gradually. In fact, many women are quite shocked by the 'bolt out of the blue' they experience. As oestrogen production decreases with the peri-menopause (the time just before) and the menopause itself, notable changes include sweating (particularly at night) and hot flushes. This is because your body thermostat goes crazy. Other symptoms include irritability, poor sleep, feeling depressed, lack of sexual appetite (or an increase!), poor concentration and memory, crying spells, tension, even nightmares.

About 15 per cent of women around the world are on some sort of hormone replacement therapy (HRT). Although very successful for some women, others find it less than satisfactory, with side-affects outweighing the menopausal symptoms. Any woman approaching the menopause should read up on it (see helpful websites, below) and then consult her doctor about the most suitable treatment for her. In addition, stick to a healthy diet rich in vitamins and minerals, exercise daily, and talk to your partner about what you're going through! Long gone are the days when partners were kept in the dark. Although rare, premature menopause can occur in those in their twenties or thirties, often due to hereditary factors. Your doctor will do a thorough endocrine (hormonal) screening to rule out anything serious. That done, early menopause may be handled the same way as later menopause.

Helpful websites – www.the-bms.org (British Menopause Society); www.womens-health-concern.org (Women's Health Concern, Help Line: 01628-483-612); www.docguide.com

Ten Ways To Live To 100

1   Have sex three times a week – research shows that the so called 'super-young' have regular sex through their 70s and beyond!

2   Take Lipoci Acid and Acetyl-L-Carnitine supplements, now believed to roll back the years. These are used to boost low energy levels and treat heart disease.

3   Replace regular tea with green tea – rich in anti-oxidants, which neutralise the damaging free radicals swarming through our systems. But if you can't get hold of green tea, regular tea helps do the trick too! Three cups a day is the optimum level.

4   Drink a glass of red wine per day to prevent heart disease. They now say some white wines have the same effect. Only a glass, mind you!

5   Laugh every day – laughter helps combat stress and anxiety, and boosts the immune system. People who can laugh take the rough with the smooth. And it feels great.

6   Drink two litres of water (preferably filtered) daily to keep your system flushed.

7   Eat blueberries, prunes, raisins and apricots – all great at mopping up those free radicals. A handful of dried fruits = concentrated nutrition with phytochemicals that help prevent cancer and heart disease.

8   Eat oily fish, which is full of omega-3 fats. It is great mood food, as well as being good for the joints, protecting against heart disease and stroke, and improving brain function.

9   Use a sun block on your face regularly – even in winter. This will reduce skin ageing and help prevent skin cancers – which are rising.

10 If your job keeps you at your desk, move around and stretch every 20 minutes and get outside at least once a day. Give yourself a head massage, shake your hands and legs – keep that blood circulating!

Chocolate

When The Going Gets Tough . . .

. . . *the tough get going*, but they also know when to let go, how to inspire others, how to look after themselves and how to keep balance in their lives. Life is what you make it. And if you're dealt a 'rough' hand you may have to work that little bit harder to reach your goals and attain your dreams. But that makes it all the more worthwhile. You only need to look at the rich and famous, with all their divorces, addictions and bad behaviour, to see that money doesn't buy happiness. Sure, money makes things *easier* but, at the end of the day, all we can hope for is to be happy with ourselves and our lives. As well as absorbing the ideas, techniques and advice from the previous pages, here are a few golden rules to live by:

➢ You are a unique person – and so is everyone else! No one will look at life the way you do, feel things the same way, or want the same things. Grow by understanding and *accepting* yourself and increasing your self-esteem. And by *learning about others!*

➢ Research shows that your thinking *affects* your life! If you leave home thinking the worst will happen, feeling bad about yourself, thinking everyone else has it better – this becomes a self-fulfilling prophecy. Go out thinking things might go your way, expecting the best from others – and you might just get it!

➢ Look at the big picture . . . but don't forget to treasure the small moments in life. What you aspire to is important. You should give your best to your work and your relationships. But along the way, don't forget to appreciate the little things – the sights and sounds of a fascinating world, the smile on your child's face, the special look from your lover, a beautiful sunset. It sounds clichéd but it's not. The happiest, most fulfilled people I know are always the first *to take time* to take a breath and enjoy the whole world around them.